NURSING CRITICALLY ILL PATIENTS CONFIDENTLY

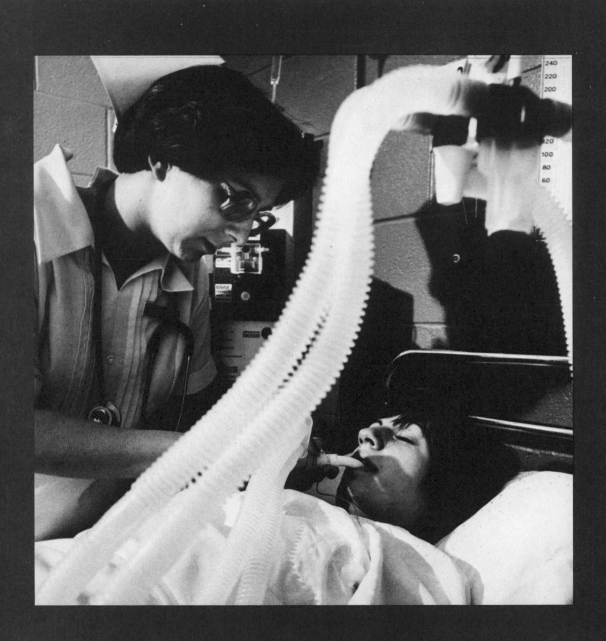

NURSING CRITICALLY ILL PATIENTS CONFIDENTLY

NURSING81 BOOKS
INTERMED COMMUNICATIONS, INC.
HORSHAM, PENNSYLVANIA

NURSING81 BOOKS, INTERMED COMMUNICATIONS, INC., HORSHAM, PENNSYLVANIA

NURSING81 BOOKS

NURSING SKILLBOOK® SERIES
Reading EKGs Correctly
Dealing with Death and Dying
Managing Diabetics Properly
Assessing Vital Functions Accurately
Helping Cancer Patients Effectively
Giving Cardiovascular Drugs Safely
Giving Emergency Care Competently
Monitoring Fluid and Electrolytes Precisely
Documenting Patient Care Responsibly
Combatting Cardiovascular Diseases Skillfully
Coping with Neurologic Problems Proficiently
Using Crisis Intervention Wisely
Nursing Critically Ill Patients Confidently

NURSING PHOTOBOOK™ SERIES
Providing Respiratory Care
Managing I.V. Therapy
Dealing with Emergencies
Giving Medications
Assessing Your Patients
Using Monitors
Providing Early Mobility
Giving Cardiac Care
Performing GI Procedures
Implementing Urologic Procedures
Controlling Infection
Giving Intensive Care
Coping with Neurologic Disorders
Caring for Surgical Patients
Managing Orthopedic Patients

Nursing81 **DRUG HANDBOOK**

Nursing80 **NURSE'S GUIDE TO DRUGS**

Nursing79 **NURSE'S GUIDE TO DRUGS**

NURSE'S REFERENCE LIBRARY

NURSING81 BOOKS
Publisher: Eugene W. Jackson
Editorial Director: Daniel L. Cheney
Graphics Director: John Isely
General Manager: T. A. Temple

NURSING SKILLBOOK® SERIES
Book Editor: Helen Hamilton
Clinical Editor: Catherine Ciaverelli Manzi, RN
Designer: Gloria J. Moyer
Marginalia Editors: Lisa Cohen, Avery Rome, Elaine Schott-Jones
Copy Editors: Pat Hamilton, Barbara Hodgson
Researcher and Indexer: Vonda Heller
Production Manager: Bernard Haas
Typography Manager: David C. Kosten
Production Assistants: Betty Mancini, Diane Paluba, Thom Staudenmayer
Artists: Robert Jackson, Robert H. Renn, Sandra Simms
Divider Art and Cover: Robert Goldstein

CLINICAL CONSULTANTS
Nancy R. Adams, RN, MSN, MAJ, ANC, *Director, Intensive Care Nursing Course Fitzsimons Army Medical Center, Denver, Colorado*
Donald De Santis, MD, *Director, Intensive Care Unit, Crozer-Chester Medical Center, Chester, Pennsylvania*
Ruth Fisher, RN, *Staff Nurse, Coronary Care Unit, Presbyterian Hospital, Philadelphia, Pennsylvania*
Bonnie Mowinski Jennings, RN, MSN, *Clinical Head Nurse, Critical Care Units, Tripler Army Medical Center, Honolulu, Hawaii*

04381

Library of Congress Cataloging in Publication Data

Main entry under title:

Nursing critically ill patients confidently.
  (Nursing Skillbook Series)
  Bibliography: p.
  Includes index.
    1. Intensive Care Nursing.   [DNLM: 1. Critical care—
Nursing texts. WY154 N974] RT120.I5N88   610.73'6
79-17515
ISBN 0-916730-13-1

CONTENTS

AUTHORS

Nancy R. Adams, one of the advisors on this book, is director of the intensive care nursing course at Fitzsimons Army Medical Center, Denver, Colorado. She received her BSN from Cornell University-New York Hospital School of Nursing, and her MSN from the Catholic University of America. She's a member of Sigma Theta Tau and the American Association of Critical Care Nurses.

Cynthia S. Butcher, a BSN graduate and MEd candidate at Michigan State University, East Lansing, is a primary care nurse at Edward W. Sparrow Hospital, Lansing, Michigan. She is a member of the Association of Nephrology Nurses and Technicians, and the American Association of Critical Care Nurses.

Christine Walton Cannon, a medical clinical specialist at Wilmington Medical Center, Delaware, received her BS from the University of Delaware, Newark, and her MSN from the University of Pennsylvania, Philadelphia. She is a member of Sigma Theta Tau, Pi Lambda Theta, and the American Association of Critical Care Nurses.

Theresa Croushore, a clinical editor for *Nursing79* Book Division, is a graduate of Saint Barnabas Hospital School of Nursing, Minneapolis, Minnesota, and a member of the Emergency Department Nurses' Association.

Patricia O'Connor Dolan is a clinical instructor of medical/surgical nursing—intensive care unit at Newton Wellesley Hospital School of Nursing in Newton, Massachusetts. A graduate of St. Elizabeth's Hospital School of Nursing in Brighton, she received her BSN and MSN from Boston University. Her memberships include Sigma Theta Tau and the American Association of Critical Care Nurses.

Shirley L. Egger graduated from St. Joseph's School of Nursing, in Hamilton, Ontario, and is a clinical teacher in the intensive care unit at Toronto Western Hospital, Ontario. She is a member of the Registered Nurses' Association of Ontario, Canada and the American Association of Critical Care Nurses.

Catherine D. Garofano, a clinical nurse in endocrinology and metabolism, and senior instructor in medicine at Hahnemann Medical College and Hospital, Philadelphia, Pennsylvania, is a graduate of St. Luke's Hospital School of Nursing, Pittsfield, Massachusetts. She received her BS from Boston University, Boston, Massachusetts.

Harry L. Greene, assistant professor of medicine, University of Massachusetts Medical Center, Worcester, is a graduate of the University of Missouri Medical School, Columbia. He served his internship and residency at Peter Bent Brigham Hospital, and a fellowship in medical oncology at Sidney Farber Cancer Center, in Boston.

Bonnie Mowinski Jennings, one of the advisors on this book, is with the U.S. Army Nurse Corps and is stationed at Tripler Army Medical Center, Honolulu, Hawaii. There, she is a clinical head nurse in the critical care units. She received her BSN and MSN at Arizona State University, Tempe, Arizona, and is a member of the Oncology Nursing Society, and the American Association of Critical Care Nurses.

Ruth Kitson, head nurse in chest surgery and medicine at Toronto Western Hospital in Ontario, Canada, is a diploma graduate of Brockville General Hospital, Ontario, and received a diploma in nursing administration from Dalhousie University in Halifax, Nova Scotia.

Marilee Molyneux Luick received her BSN from Seton Hall University College of Nursing, South Orange, New Jersey, where she is presently working on her MSN. She is an inservice instructor at Jersey Shore Medical Center, Neptune, New Jersey, an advanced life support instructor for the New Jersey Heart Association, and a member of the American Association of Critical Care Nurses.

Edwina A. McConnell is clinical director of surgical nursing at Madison General Hospital in Madison, Wisconsin. She received her BSN from Boston University in Boston, and her MSN from the University of Colorado, Denver. She is a member of the American Nurses' Association, Sigma Theta Tau, and the A.M.W.A.

R. R. Rich is a nurse clinician in the critical care unit, Massachusetts General Hospital, Boston. She received her BSN at Duquesne University, Pittsburgh, and her MSN at Catholic University of America.

Hannelore M. Sweetwood is inservice director at Jersey Shore Medical Center, Neptune, New Jersey. A graduate of Jersey City Medical Center School of Nursing, she received her BS from Monmouth College, West Long Branch, where she is working on her master's degree.

Karen E. Witt received her BSN and MSN from the University of Wisconsin, Madison, and is an instructor at the University of Wisconsin School of Nursing in Eau Claire. She's a member of the American Nurses' Association and the Wisconsin Nurses' Association.

FOREWORD

What's special about caring for patients who are critically ill? Nursing is fundamentally the same for every patient. But when the patient is critically ill—when his vital functions are so dangerously unstable that he can deteriorate radically from one moment to the next—he needs your nursing skills tuned to perfection: observation that's supersharp, alert to the tiniest change; attention to detail that's totally precise; and the ability to make irreversible decisions quickly and correctly. Such highly skilled care may be given in a specially designed intensive care unit. But, depending on circumstances and on the facilities available in your community, you may be called upon to give it on the regular medical/surgical floor.

Wherever it's given, such lifesaving competence always rests on a foundation of knowledge. Before you can competently take care of a person who's critically ill, you must understand the relationships between body systems—how and why they fail and how abnormalities in one system quickly spread to the others. You must know which diseases and conditions most often produce critical illness; what symptoms to look for; what laboratory methods confirm their presence or response to treatment; what treatment methods are effective against them; and what their effects and possible complications are.

This Skillbook, *Nursing Critically Ill Patients Confidently*, can give you such knowledge and can help you to improve the quality of your nursing skills. In its 13 chapters, nurse specialists share their extensive clinical experience in caring for patients who are critically ill. They review a reliable method for bedside assessment; summarize problems peculiar to the intensive care unit; tell how to cope with critical illness that reflects failure of the vital systems—cardiovascular, respiratory, renal, neurologic, hepatic, and endocrine; and describe management of postoperative recovery and of disseminated intravascular clotting (DIC). Throughout, they summarize symptoms and physical signs, laboratory examinations (including normal lab values and abnormal values and how they relate to certain system failures), and current treatment methods. They offer step-by-step instructions for using special procedures and special equipment. And they put all the information together for you in detailed case histories.

This Skillbook can help you to grow in competence and confidence and, so, enhance the quality of nursing care you give critically ill patients.

—LENETTE OWENS BURRELL, RN, BS,
MSN, EdD
Associate Professor
Medical College of Georgia, School of Nursing
Athens, Georgia
Coauthor of the Textbook,
Critical Care—3rd edition
C. V. Mosby Co., St. Louis, 1977

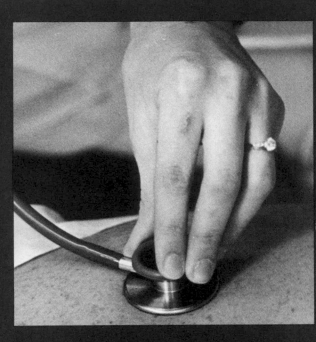
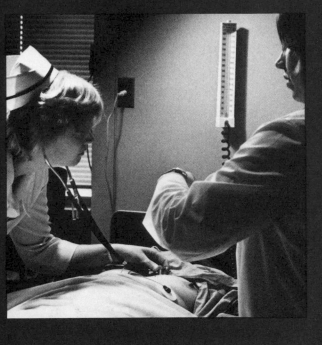
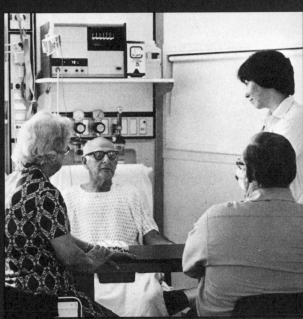
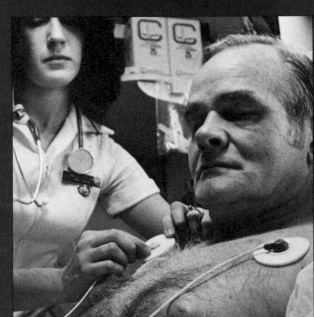

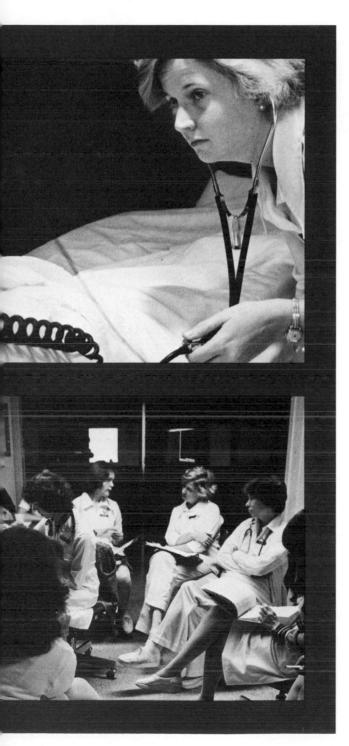

COPING WITH CRITICAL ILLNESS

1

INITIAL ASSESSMENT
Acquiring a nursing baseline

BY RUTH KITSON, RN

YOUR INITIAL ASSESSMENT of the critically ill patient provides your baseline for planning and implementing nursing care. If your assessment is inaccurate or incomplete, the nursing care that follows can be inadequate, inappropriate, and, perhaps, even unsafe. Naturally, this first assessment in a person who is desperately ill must be brief until his condition has stabilized. If on first seeing the patient, you realize his airway is not patent, the *only* action you should take is to establish a patent airway and stabilize his respiratory status. In a severely distressed patient, the ABCs of critical care nursing always apply:

• Establish a patent Airway.
• Be sure the patient is Breathing.
• Check for adequate Circulation.

Once the patient's cardiorespiratory status has stabilized, you can continue with thorough, system-by-system assessment. Before going into the details of system assessment, let's review some general principles about it. First of all, just what is assessment? Actually, it's the process that requires you to make a judgment about a patient's condition; it takes in the sum total of what you conclude about his state of health. You can arrive at this conclusion in many ways. But it always begins with your visual impression. Drawing on your past experience, you can often identify some conditions, almost at a glance. For example, you quickly suspect respiratory failure when you notice restlessness, tachycardia, diaphoresis, nasal flaring, use of accessory intercostal muscles, poor chest expansion and depressed respirations. And, if you're a nurse with a lot of clinical experience, your assessment is sometimes influenced by a "sixth" sense — not very scientific but, nonetheless, amazingly reliable.

If you're like me, you've often said, without a speck of hard evidence — "Mr. X looks like he's going into shock" — and found him in clinical shock a short time later. So trust your instinct. Follow up on these subliminal clues, which can alert you to look for important changes in the patient's condition. For example, if you suspect shock, monitor vital signs more frequently until you're sure he's stable and inform the doctor.

Two sources: Three methods
What are your sources of information for an accurate assessment? There are two: The first or "primary" source is the patient. The second, called the "secondary" source, includes information from all other sources: other people, the patient's family, health records, and so forth. You can obtain information from these sources by three methods: 1) the patient's history—a description of the patient's chief complaints, a patient profile, present problems, and past health history (including a family health history); 2) thorough physical examination; 3) baseline laboratory data.

Take a complete history
Begin with the patient's chief complaint, as he himself describes it. For example, he may say he's been extremely short of breath for the last two days. Always ask how long he's had this symptom, what brings it on, and what relieves it. Record the symptom using the patient's own words to describe it.

Thoroughly analyze the patient's chief symptom. Find out when it started; if its onset was gradual or sudden; and if something unusual (such as infection or fatigue) precipitated it. Find out everything you can about the symptom's characteristics. Its location, severity, pattern of occurrence, and any associated symptoms are all important to your assessment. Is the symptom new, or had it occurred before? If so, has the

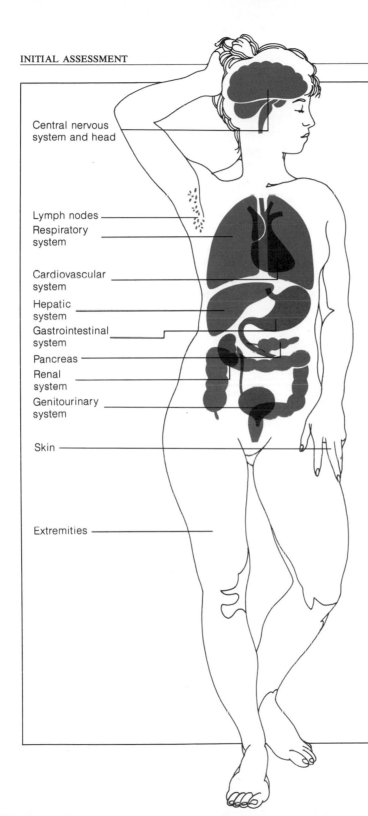

Central nervous
system and head

Lymph nodes

Respiratory
system

Cardiovascular
system

Hepatic
system

Gastrointestinal
system

Pancreas

Renal
system

Genitourinary
system

Skin

Extremities

Head to toe

To avoid missing important data, once you've assessed the patient's present condition, carefully review all body systems from head to toe. What might turn up?

● *Central nervous system and head:* dizziness, headache, convulsions, paralysis, loss of conciousness.
● *Eyes:* visual problems, pain, infection.
● *Nose and sinuses:* epistaxis, discharge, deformities, obstruction.
● *Ears:* discharge, earaches, hearing problems, tinnitus.
● *Mouth:* bleeding gums, hoarseness, toothache.
● *Neck:* enlarged thyroid gland, pain.
● *Nodes:* palpable axillary nodes, tenderness.
● *Respiratory:* wheezing, rales, shortness of breath.
● *Cardiovascular:* angina, hypertension, heart murmur, history of coronary artery disease.
● *Gastrointestinal:* indigestion, constipation, diarrhea, history of GI pain or ulcers.
● *Genitourinary:* hematuria, frequent urination.
● *Renal:* flank pain, renal calculi.
● *Liver:* tenderness, enlargement, history of cirrhosis.
● *Extremities:* varicose veins, intermittent claudication; fractures, pain.
● *Skin:* rash, delayed wound healing, tendency to bruise.
● *Endocrine:* diabetes, hypoglycemia, unusual growth history.
● *Allergies:* allergy to food, medication, or immunization.
● *Immunizations:* date of last tetanus immunization.

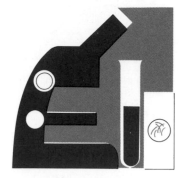

Normal lab values
ELECTROLYTES
Sodium (Na): 136 to 145 mEq/L
Potassium (K): 3.5 to 5.0 mEq/L
Calcium (Ca): 8.8 to 10.5 mg/100
    ml or 4.5 to 5.5 mEq/L
Magnesium (Mg): 1.5 to 2.5 mEq/L
Chloride (Cl): 95 to 109 mEq/L

BUN: 10-20 mg/100 ml
Serum bilirubin (total): 0.1 to 1.2
    mg/dl
Creatinine: 0.5 to 1.5 mg/100 ml

COMPLETE BLOOD COUNT
White blood cells (WBC): 4500 to
    11,000/microliter (ul)
Red blood cells (RBC):
    Male, 4.6 to 6.2 x 10⁶/ul
    Female, 4.2 to 5.4 x 10⁶/ul
Hemoglobin (Hgb): Male: 13.5
    to 18.0 g/dl
    Female: 12.0 to 16.0 g/dl

(continued)

patient had recurring episodes, or is it continuous? Has it changed in any way? Is it more or less severe?

After you have carefully analyzed the patient's present symptoms, do a thorough review of *systems*. This will help eliminate the possibility of overlooking important data. Do this in a systematic way, preferably from head to toe, so you don't forget anything. Such a review might turn up information like the following:

• Skin: lesions, bruising, dryness, delayed wound healing
• Head: injury, headache, dizziness
• Eyes: infection, pain, vision problems
• Ears: earaches, poor hearing, occasional discharge
• Nose and sinuses: epistaxis, nasal obstruction, discharge
• Mouth: toothache, bleeding gums, hoarseness
• Neck: pain, enlarged thyroid
• Nodes: tenderness, axillary nodes
• Breast: pain, tenderness, operation for cysts
• Respiratory: chest pain, wheezing, stridor, dyspnea, pneumonia, bronchitis
• Cardiovascular: cyanosis, history of heart murmur, coronary artery disease, hypertension, last EKG
• Gastrointestinal: constipation, diarrhea, melenic stools, jaundice, dyspepsia
• Genitourinary: renal colic, frequency of urination, hematuria, abnormal menstrual history
• Extremities: varicose veins, intermittent claudication, fractures, pain
• Back: morning stiffness, limitation of movement
• Central nervous system: loss of consciousness, convulsions, speech disorders, weakness, paralysis
• Hematopoietic: bleeding gums, anemia
• Endocrine: diabetes, hypoglycemia, unusual growth history
• Allergies: penicillin, food
• Immunizations: date last tetanus injection.

Patient profile important
Be sure to include a patient profile (a description of the patient's personal background and life-style). This is very important since his illness will probably influence his daily living patterns. Find out the patient's personal history. Include his age, birthplace, marital status, education, race, and occupation. You can see how important this information can be if

you look at the following example: A 50-year-old man was hospitalized because his shortness of breath had become increasingly worse over the last several weeks. He had worked in the coal mines for over 30 years. These few facts alone suggest the right diagnosis: mine-workers' pneumoconiosis (black lung disease).

Your records should include the patient's life pattern: his sleep habits (number of hours per day); diet; exercise; alcohol and tobacco intake; present medications; source of income and his living environment. Knowing these things can help you plan comprehensive care and make hospitalization a less disruptive experience. A critical part of the patient's profile is his family history: their current health; their independence of or dependence on the patient; their occupations; their ages; how the patient's illness affects them; how they interact with him; and how they can help him during his illness.

A history as detailed as this takes some time to complete. You may obtain it from his family if the patient is too sick to answer questions, or you may wait and discuss this with him as soon as he is able. In either case, you'll complete the detailed history sometime *after* the physical examination.

Give a thorough exam

As you know, a thorough physical examination has four essential parts: inspection, palpation, percussion, and auscultation. Physical examination always begins with *inspection*. The "at-a-glance" assessment mentioned above is a good starting point, but always support your first impressions with a studied, deliberate, visual examination. Look carefully at the patient and record the physical characteristics you find. For example, when inspecting his thorax, notice the shape of his chest and any abnormalities of his sternum, spine, or ribs. Expect chest expansion to be equal bilaterally. Any inequalities in chest expansion may indicate a pneumothorax or flail chest. Notice the patient's respiratory rate, and its depth and pattern. Does he have a cough? If so, describe it, and the amount and characteristics of any sputum. For example, pink, frothy sputum may indicate pulmonary edema. Purulent sputum (yellow, green, grey) is suggestive of pneumonia or bronchitis.

During *palpation*, you may be able to identify temperature abnormalities, vibrations, pulsations, tenderness, swelling,

Normal lab values (continued)
Hematocrit (Hct): 37 to 47 ml/100 ml
Platelets: 140,000 to 440,000/cu mm of blood
Prothrombin time (PT): 12-14 sec.
Partial thromboplastin time (PTT): 60-70 sec.
Coagulation time: 9-12 min. (Lee White method)
Fasting blood sugar (FBS): 60-100 mg/100 ml

ARTERIAL BLOOD GAS (ABG)
pH: 7.35 to 7.45
PO_2: 80-100 mm Hg
PCO_2: 34-46 mm Hg
HCO_3: 22-26 mEq/L
Base excess: -2 to +2
O_2 saturation: 95%

URINALYSIS
Specific gravity: 1.010 to 1.030
pH: 4.6 to 8.0 (average 6.0)
Color: yellow, clear
Glucose, protein, casts, RBCs, crystals: negative

OSMOLARITY
Serum: 280 to 294 mOsm/Kg
Urine: 50 to 1200 mOsm/L
SGOT: 8-33U/ml
Cholesterol: 150 to 250 mg/dl (varies with diet and age)

CEREBROSPINAL FLUID (CSF)
Albumin: 10 to 30 mg/dl
Calcium: 2.1 to 2.9 mEq/L
Cell count: 0 to 8 cells/ul
Chloride: 118 to 132 mEq/L
Glucose: 45 to 75 mg/dl
Protein (total): 15-45 mg/dl

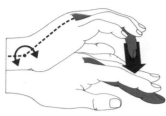

Telltale taps
Percussion helps you assess the size, position, and density of internal organs. With your hands placed over the area to examine, strike the middle phalanx of the middle finger of one hand with the middle finger of your other hand, as shown above. The sound produced can tell you whether the organ is filled with air or fluid. Study the list of percussion sounds below to help you improve your percussion technique.
Flat: soft intensity, high pitch, short duration, as in thigh
Dull: medium intensity, medium pitch, medium duration, as in liver
Resonant: loud intensity, low pitch, long duration, as in normal lung
Hyperresonant: very loud intensity, lower pitch, longer duration, as in emphysemic lung
Tympanic: loud, bell-like intensity, variable pitch, variable duration, as in gastric air bubble.

rigidity, and so forth. Palpation may confirm information acquired during inspection. It's especially useful for examining the chest. For example, you may feel a crackling beneath the skin that indicates subcutaneous emphysema or air in tissues (as in pneumothorax). Also, if you hold your hands against both sides of the patient's chest while he repeatedly says "99", you may be able to detect the increased vibrations of pleural effusion.

With *percussion,* you can determine the density of an organ or tissue by the quality of the vibration elicited by tapping it. For example, percussion over the stomach should elicit the hollow sound of a gas-filled organ.

Auscultation, of course, is the study of sounds you can hear with a stethoscope. You're well aware of its use in identifying abnormal heart sounds. However, remember to use it for evaluating breath sounds too. In patients with asthma or bronchitis, you'll often hear rhonchi. These wheezing, whistling, musical sounds are usually heard on expiration. They're due to shortening or narrowing of the airway from bronchospasm or heavy secretions. Rales are short, bubbly sounds generally heard on inspiration. As air is drawn into the lungs, any secretions that have collected along the walls are pulled in the same direction causing the bubbly sound.

Auscultation may also help you recognize atelectasis (collapse of alveoli in local or generalized areas). Recognize it by the decreased intensity or absence of breath sounds. Also listen for a pleural rub — a coarse, creaky sound heard at the end of inspiration and the beginning of expiration. It results from friction when inflamed surfaces of the pleura rub together (as in pleurisy). You can usually hear this pleural rub in the lower areas of the chest wall.

A thorough physical examination is crucial for implementing appropriate care and for establishing a baseline for measuring the patient's improvement or deterioration.

Laboratory tests routine
Every critically ill patient needs certain laboratory and diagnostic tests to confirm and supplement the physical findings. For example, a urinalysis and complete blood count are routine and essential. Urinalysis often reveals glycosuria. Depending on the patient's illness, other routine tests may include electrolytes, blood urea nitrogen (BUN), blood sugar,

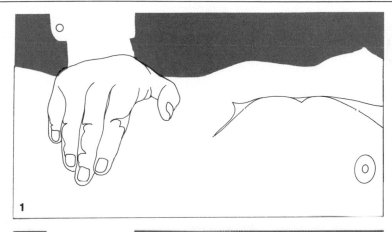

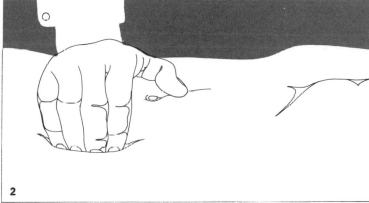

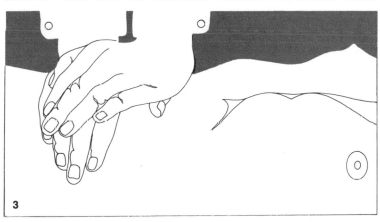

Press toward the mark

In palpation you examine a relaxed, supine patient by feeling and pressing his abdomen with your palms and fingers (Fig. 1). Once you have mastered this technique, you should be able to discern the position, size, and resistance of organs, and reveal pain, tenderness, or any unidentifiable masses.

You can perform *light palpation* by placing your palm on the patient's abdomen and pressing your fingertips gently into the abdominal wall (Fig. 2). Make sure your hands are warm so you don't make the patient tense. Palpate the entire area as the patient breathes first normally and then deeply.

In *deep palpation* (Fig. 3), you use the entire palm of one hand to press deeply into the abdomen or you can place one hand on top of the other and press in the manner shown at left.

Assessment guidelines
Obtain the following information
from your patient on admission or
as soon as possible.

CHIEF COMPLAINT: As patient sees
it.

DURATION OF ILLNESS: As patient
recalls, has it affected his
life-style?

MEDICAL HISTORY: Previous
hospitalizations? Reason? When?
Results? Lab and diagnostic
studies?

OBSERVATION OF PATIENT'S
CONDITION: Level of
consciousness? Well-nourished?
Healthy? Skin color, integrity, and
turgor? Senses? Headaches?
Cough? Syncope? Nausea?
Convulsions? Edema? Lumps?
Bruises? Bleeding?
Inflammation? Pressure areas?
Range of motion? Unusual
sensations? Pain? Vital signs?

MENTAL AND EMOTIONAL STATUS:
Cooperative? Anxious?
Language difficulties?
Understanding of his condition
and expectations? Ask what the
doctor told him. Mood?
Self-image? Reaction to stress?
Rapport with interviewer and
staff? Compatibility with
roommate?

ALLERGIES: Food? Drugs? Type of
reaction?

MEDICATION: Dosage? Why
taken? When taken? Last dose?
(continued)

SGOT, SMA-12, hemoglobin, hematocrit, WBC and platelet count. Also routine in almost every critically ill patient — a preliminary electrocardiogram to serve as a cardiovascular baseline, and a chest X-ray. Chest X-rays often reveal certain problems that require immediate attention such as pneumothorax, pleural effusion, ruptured diaphragm, or lung shadows. Blood-gas analysis is indicated for any patient likely to have respiratory distress; coagulation studies for a patient with suspected bleeding problems (see Chapter 13).

Keep track of vital signs

In a patient who's critically ill, vital signs are much more than an index of present condition. They may also suggest trends or forecast changes. So your meticulous assessment of vital signs can sometimes help prevent needless complications. Take the patient's *temperature* as soon as possible to record a baseline. The oral temperature is most desirable. But if the patient is confused, comatose, or receiving oxygen, a rectal temperature is preferable. Keep in mind that a patient who is just developing a fever may feel cool to the touch (superficial blood vessels are constricted to conserve heat and skin may be pale and mottled). He may feel cold to the point of rigor (sometimes with continuous, uncontrolled shaking). However, soon after this stage, the body temperature goes up with all the usual manifestations of fever. Remember that in a critically ill patient, a sudden fever over 102.2° F. (39° C.) with chills, malaise, confusion, fast deep breathing, tachycardia and a sudden drop in systolic pressure (to 80 or below), often indicate septic shock.

When taking the patient's pulse, remember to compare the radial and apical pulses (taken simultaneously) — that'll tell you more about cardiac efficiency than the radial pulse alone. For example, a marked difference between apical and radial pulses could indicate atrial fibrillation. A markedly rapid pulse (over 110 beats per minute) may indicate hypoxic shock due to reduced cardiac output, blood loss, pulmonary embolism, or some other gross physiologic insult. Take a critically ill patient's pulse for at least a full minute to detect any rhythmic irregularities or ectopic beats and also observe the cardiac monitor frequently.

Watch the quality and pattern of *respirations*. You can't watch respirations too carefully in patients who are critically ill. Normal respirations should be relaxed, effortless, and regular (normal rate, 12 to 18 breaths per minute). Normally, the diaphragm assists respiration. If you see that a patient needs to use intercostal or accessory muscles in his neck to help him breathe, he's developing respiratory failure. Dyspnea (difficult, labored breathing) may suggest pulmonary embolism, pneumothorax, or left-sided heart failure.

Measuring the patient's *blood pressure* is as important as it is commonplace. Remember that one reading may not be significant; a series of readings is usually more informative and reliable. However, if the initial blood pressure is 160/90 and the next reading is 100/70, you can safely suspect impending shock. Falling blood pressure reflects reduced output or reduced peripheral vessel resistance. Be sure to record both systolic and diastolic pressures. (The systolic pressure indicates the maximum exertion against the arteries by the left ventricle; diastolic pressure indicates blood vessel resistance.) Evaluating the pulse pressure is also important.

When you have completed your data after taking the patient's temperature, pulse, respirations, and blood pressure, combine it with the patient's history, laboratory findings, and physical examination for a thorough and accurate assessment. Let's see how this procedure for assessment worked in one critically ill patient:

Mr. Wolfson, a 43-year-old construction worker, was brought in by the rescue squad after falling 15 feet at work. He had severe pain in his chest (over his lateral and anterior left rib cage). He was in great distress and couldn't give a history. Since none of his family or friends were present to give a history either, the physical examination began immediately.

Inspection showed a patent airway. He was breathing adequately to maintain sufficient ventilation and circulation. However, a careful look at his chest showed marked indrawing of the left chest wall during inspiration (flail chest).

While palpating his chest, the examiner felt a crackling under the skin in the left side (subcutaneous emphysema) which raised the possibility of a pneumothorax. This was later confirmed. Palpation also revealed extreme tenderness in the anterior left side below the diaphragm. Auscultation revealed an absence of breath sounds in the lower left base of the lung and rales throughout the rest of the lung field. An immediate chest X-ray showed fractured ribs (from 4 to 12) on the left side

Assessment guidelines
(continued)
Does he have it with him? Any other drugs taken occasionally? Recently? Why? OTC drugs?

PROSTHESES: Pacemaker? Trach? Drainage tubes? Feeding tube? Catheter? Ostomy appliance? Breast form? Hearing aid? Glasses or contacts? Dentures? Cane? Walker? Brace? False eye? Prosthetic leg?

REVIEW OF SYSTEMS: Cardiopulmonary, neurologic, renal, etc.

PERSONAL BEHAVIOR PATTERNS: *Sleep:* When? Aids? Difficulties? *Activity:* Self-care? Daily exercise? Ambulatory? *Elimination patterns:* Continent? Frequency? Nocturia? Characteristics of stool/urine? Pain? Discharge? *Diet:* Feeds self? Diet restrictions (therapeutic, cultural, preferential)? Frequency? Snacks? Alcohol? Fad diets? *Health practices:* Breast self-exam? Physical exam? *Life-style:* Parents? Family? Children? Residence? Occupation? Personal hygiene? Recreation? Interests? Financial status? Religion? Education? Ethnic background?

TYPICAL DAY PROFILE: Have patient describe how he spends his time.

INFORMANT: From whom did you obtain this information? Patient? Family? Old records? Ambulance driver?

and a large pneumothorax. A chest tube (#26) was inserted immediately and connected to an Emerson suction machine.

Blood-gas analysis results were: pH 7.28; PO_2 54; PCO_2 70. Mr. Wolfson was clearly in respiratory failure, and was immediately intubated for ventilation with an MA-1 ventilator, to correct his blood gases and stabilize his flail chest.

At this time, a *stat* EKG showed no abnormality other than a sinus tachycardia. Blood workup included hemoglobin, hematocrit, WBC, SMA-12, BUN, and blood sugar. The hemoglobin was 8.6%, suggesting a ruptured spleen. Vital signs were to be monitored every 15 minutes until his condition stabilized and he could be taken to surgery for splenectomy.

In the meantime, Mr. Wolfson's family arrived and helped with the completion of his history and personal profile. They told us that he was married, and had six children. He and his family lived in an expensive new home on which he was having problems maintaining payments. He began taking diazepam (Valium) for anxiety that was mainly due to financial worries.

With the patient's family available to answer questions, we were able to complete a thorough, system-by-system review and medical history. The patient's skin, head, eyes, ears, nose, oral cavity, neck and nodes were normal. He had a history of asthma in childhood, but had had no symptoms since he was 6 years old. His cardiovascular system was apparently normal. He had no history of hypertension or heart murmurs. He had a 2-year history of gastric ulcers that had become more severe recently. However, they had been controlled with diet. He had no history of back trouble. His back showed no limitation of movement other than that caused by the fractured ribs and flail chest. As far as could be determined, he had not lost consciousness during the fall and had no speech disorder or paralysis. His falling hemoglobin was corrected by a splenectomy and four units of packed cells intravenously. He had no thyroid or other endocrine problems.

The above assessment and beginning treatment took place over approximately 6 hours and included a physical examination and routine laboratory workup.

Clearly, your assessment of a critically ill patient is complex. It must be accurate and, often, it must be fast — because such a patient's condition can deteriorate drastically in just a few minutes. Fortunately, such assessment is not too difficult if you follow a systematic and thorough approach.

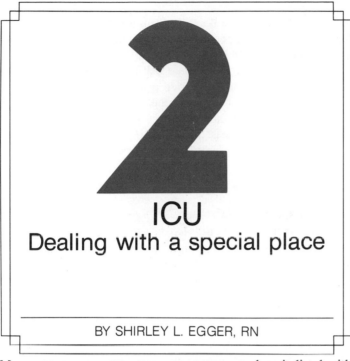

ICU
Dealing with a special place

BY SHIRLEY L. EGGER, RN

MR. RUSSELL, A 29-YEAR-OLD TEACHER, was hospitalized with pneumonia only 24 hours ago. Now, because of impending respiratory failure and the need for careful monitoring and assisted ventilation, he's been transferred to the intensive care unit (ICU).

ICU. Just the word itself conjures up a variety of mental images. To Mr. Russell, the ICU may seem like a bizarre collection of sensations and procedures that continually intrude on a lonely inner world dominated by fear and the struggle to breathe. To his wife, the complicated equipment, bright lighting, and efficiently starched personnel may seem as foreign (and as frightening) as a scene from a science fiction movie. And to you, the nurse, the ICU may seem like the top—the realm of a competitive, highly motivated elite. Because the ICU is a very special place it can present special problems for all who come into contact with it. First, let's look more closely at how the ICU affects the patient.

The ICU patient: Triply stressed
A week ago, Mr. Russell seemed fairly healthy, except for a slight cold. He and his wife had just bought a new home, and

Keeping the lid on infection
The average ICU patient has at least 3 invasive procedures daily—placing a PA line, an arterial line, a catheter—the list goes on. These procedures raise the risk of infection, which could prove fatal in someone already critically ill. To prevent such infection:
• Be especially careful when flushing, inserting, or removing a catheter, or other invasive devices.
• Wash your hands frequently, not just between patients, but between procedures as well. This can prevent the transfer of bacteria from one part of the body to another.
• Keep your hair cut short or tied back. Don't wear rings or nail polish, since these can harbor bacteria.
• Have lotions, soaps, hand creams, and other liquids that may act as a culture medium tested periodically for bacteria. Also, keep these liquids tightly covered.
• Have frequent bacteriology checks of the whole unit.
• Set up and stick to a regular housekeeping schedule.
• Keep visitors and staff with obvious infections off the unit. And don't let the ICU become a thoroughfare or sideshow for other hospital personnel, or nursing or medical students.
• Use reverse isolation in patients with low white blood cell counts.
    Some recently built ICUs are divided into small cubicles to reduce the infection rate. Some even go a step further—and have a completely separate isolation room.

their two children were doing well in nursery school and kindergarten. Suddenly, he was struck with an acute illness. Now, Mr. Russell lies fighting for every breath. An X-ray technician tries to shove a cold X-ray plate behind his back. One nurse stabs an artery to study his blood gases, while another insists that he try to expectorate. On top of all this, he's coping with fear—this isn't just the hospital, it's the ICU. He wonders how bad his condition really is…if he's going to die…how his wife is…how she'll manage with him away from home and out of work.

According to one psychiatrist, psychologic stress is caused by:
• loss of something of value
• injury or threat of bodily harm, or
• frustration of drive.
By this definition, the critically ill ICU patient is triply stressed, and he's forced to deal with this stress while coping with an illness that taxes his very ability to do so.

Mr. Russell *has* clearly lost things of value to any human being: his independence, his privacy, his ability to care for himself. His role as husband, father, and teacher are all circumscribed. He's been intubated; he can't speak and can't express his fear and frustration. His urinary output is monitored by an indwelling catheter; most of his other bodily functions are also monitored. He's forced to wear skimpy clothing and lies separated from his neighbor by a thin curtain—nothing more.

He's fearful about his physical condition: Will a nurse accidentally jostle him and make his breathing even more painful? What if the ventilator he's connected to gives out?

And his drive is frustrated: When will he be able to go back to work? How will his wife manage by herself in their new house?

Whirrs, bubbles, hisses, and beeps
Besides these stresses, the ICU patient also experiences sensory overload. There's the constant soft whirring of a fan, the bubbling of oxygen through water, the hissing of oxygen valves, or the gentle beeping of the monitor. The lights, more often than not, continually shine brightly. Hospital personnel are constantly prodding, probing, or otherwise disturbing him. All this—on top of the constant discomfort he may feel from tubes

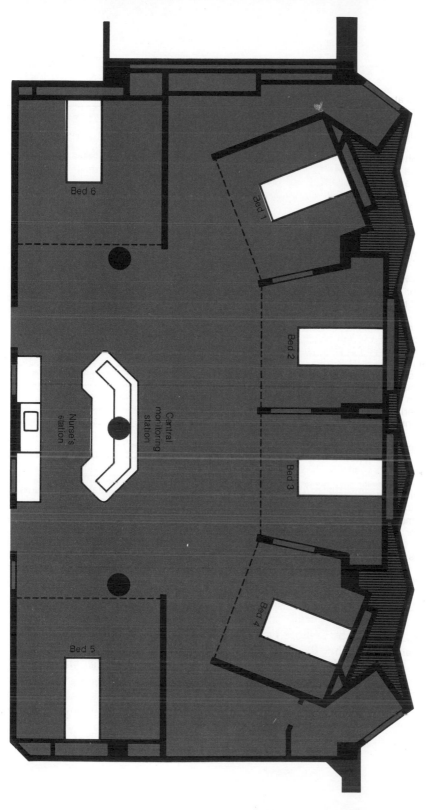

PLANNING FOR PRIVACY

To ensure patient privacy and help reduce infection, the ICU may be divided into cubicles as shown here. The open end of the room may be covered with a curtain during certain procedures, but otherwise it's left open so the patient can be seen from the nursing station.

Using a sawtooth-designed windowed outside wall gives every patient a view without blocking your view of the patients. And placing each cubicle at an angle increases bed capacity.

The unit may be divided into two areas—the closest for the most acutely ill patients and the remainder for patients whose care is less complex.

Bed 6

Bed 1

Bed 2

Bed 3

Bed 4

Bed 5

Nurse's station

Central monitoring station

A GOOD NIGHT'S SLEEP

Delta waves which are very slow and high mark the start of stage 4 sleep.

R.E.M., final sleep cycle, waves show an active EEG.

Normal sleep is a cyclical process which consists of 4 stages of increasing depth: 1, 2, 3, 4. One complete sleep cycle lasts from 80 to 120 minutes.

Rapid eye movement (REM) sleep occurs as the sleeper emerges from the deepest stage. As its name implies, REM sleep is characterized by rapid movement of the eyes, and is associated with dreaming.

REM sleep is the restorative phase of sleep. It appears to be needed for the release of psychologic tension, and for effective adaption to physical and emotional surroundings during our waking hours. REM sleep is needed in greater quantities after stress or worry. Even partial deprivation of sleep (especially REM sleep) can impair memory and mental agility, limit the attention span, and induce hallucinations, and temporary neurosis or psychosis. After a period of sleep deprivation, normal mental function may not return for as long as 10 days. To help patients get the sleep they need:

• Cluster treatments and family visits as much as possible without overtaxing patients, to allow for longer periods of rest in between.

• Encourage naps in the morning rather than the afternoon. Morning naps are mostly a continuation of REM sleep, and usually leave patients feeling more refreshed. Also, if patients nap in the morning instead of the afternoon, they're apt to sleep better at night.

• Find out what your patients' sleep routines were at home, and try to let them follow them as much as possible. Certain rituals, such as a bedtime snack, or familiar objects, such as a favorite pillow may help promote sleep.

• At night, make sure unit lights are dimmed and unnecessary lights are out. Be quiet and avoid unnecessary noisy procedures.

• Turn off the nurses' station radio at night, or turn it down so patients can't hear it.

• After establishing a successful sleep plan for a specific patient, record it so it can be followed again.

• If anxiety is keeping a patient awake, put him in touch with the hospital social worker or other personnel who can help alleviate worry.

• Unless they're absolutely necessary, avoid giving sedatives. While these drugs induce sleep, they may also alter the normal sleep cycle.

and dressings, and the pain caused by his physical condition.

In other ways, the ICU patient experiences sensory deprivation, which can cause psychologic disturbances and even hallucinations. The white, sterile ICU may lack windows. The patient's vision may be blurred because his eyeglasses have been taken away to make room for tubes or dressings; his hearing may be dulled because his hearing aid's been removed. He lies immobile, staring at the harsh whiteness of the ceiling over his head.

The 24-hour lighting eliminates his sense of day and night. He may lose his sense of time altogether, because of the lack of clocks or normal sleeping and eating routines. Because of constant interruptions, noise, and the bright lights, the ICU patient rarely completes even one sleep cycle (from 80 to 120 minutes). Some researchers have postulated that this sleep deprivation may be at least partially to blame for the ICU patient's delirious, catastrophic, or euphoric response: These are responses to the environment, as well as the illness. To help him sleep, the patient may be sedated. This, too, can lead to psychologic disturbances.

Second childhood

The ICU patient is encouraged to regress through his illness; to become like a child again. All his needs are taken care of, and this may impede his assuming responsibility once he does get better.

A critically ill person may feel he's expected to be irritable and may use this opportunity to express pent-up aggression that was carefully hidden when he was well. The patient who normally shirks responsibility at last may have found an acceptable way to do so. Family relationships may change: A domineering husband may be made helpless, to his wife's satisfaction; a submissive wife may use her illness to get her way.

The ICU patient often tries to express himself through behavior, perhaps because he can't speak, or to regain some control over his life, or to prove to himself that he's well. Too often the staff's response is to restrain him immediately and to label him as uncooperative, which increases his confinement and his anxiety.

What can you do?

The picture of the ICU patient I've painted above does seem pretty bleak, but you can do a lot to improve it. Perhaps one of the simplest ways is to initiate small changes in the ICU to help make it less foreboding. Try to avoid restraining the patient, if possible. Ask the patient's family to bring in small objects from home that he'll recognize. To lessen sensory deprivation, let him wear his eyeglasses, dentures, or hearing aid, if he's able.

Mobiles hung from the ceiling can brighten the ICU for everyone and can be easily seen even by patients who are immobile. If your unit has windows (many ICUs don't, for some odd reason), try to place the beds so the patients have a view. Provide some sense of time by hanging calendars and clocks on the walls where patients can see them. Turning the lights down or off at night can be a big help in reestablishing normal diurnal rhythms and can also help the ICU patient get the sleep he so desperately needs. Keep monitors, respirators, and other noisy equipment away from the patient's head. Try to space patient care to allow for rest between procedures and for longer periods of uninterrupted sleep. Scheduling care at planned intervals can also give the patient something definite to look forward to and can help establish some sense of time. Instead of adhering to a strict 5-minutes-per-hour visiting schedule, try letting the family visit directly before or after care—when you'll be interrupting the patient's rest anyway.

People, not things
Although the ICU, by nature, doesn't allow for much patient privacy or dignity, do what you can to make the patient feel less like an object. Don't talk about him at his bedside, unless he's included in these conferences. Handle his personal belongings with extra care—these are the only things in the ICU he can call his own, so they take on special meaning for him. Taking the time to stop and talk, or even to just be near the patient, is extremely important. Touching the patient's hand gently as you ask questions can help show him that you care. Don't forget to introduce yourself before you touch a patient and to talk to him about the care as you give it, even if he's comatose or doesn't seem to respond. We've all probably had the experience of caring for a comatose patient, even of talking about him at his bedside, as if he didn't exist, only to have him tell us later exactly what had gone on around him. Try not to fall into this trap.

Mr. Russell is not the "pneumonia on the ventilator" or a series of chest X-rays or blood-gas results. The complicated ICU gadgetry can distract you, but resist the temptation of thinking of patients and treating them as objects connected to this machinery. The best ICU nurse sees her patient first, the patient's condition second, and the equipment last.

If the patient can't talk but can communicate, give him a magic slate, an alphabet board, or a clipboard, paper, and pencil, and encourage him to use it. If possible, try phrasing questions to allow for a simple yes or no answer. Use every opportunity to observe the patient's mental status, as well as his physical condition. If a patient seems depressed, try to get him to think of the future, rather than the not-very-pleasant present. Tell him when his family or friends call with a message, and keep him aware of news and sports events—anything to get his mind off his illness. If a patient acts too independent, he's probably frightened of the helplessness he feels. Try to

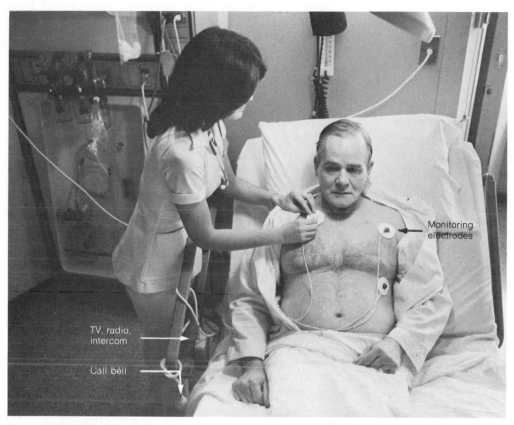

Monitoring electrodes

TV, radio, intercom

Call bell

Shock of your life
Because of the vast array of electrical equipment in the ICU, electrical accidents are a real danger. To prevent them:
• Check electrical cords often. Make sure the insulation isn't cracked or frayed. Keep the cords away from heat and from sharp, greasy, or wet surfaces. Check that electrical plugs and outlets aren't loose or broken.
• Make sure all electrical equipment is grounded. (It should have a 3-pronged plug.)
• Be able to identify equipment malfunctions. If a machine gives you a slight shock, or if it sparks, smokes, or overheats, notify the proper authorities, and disconnect the equipment if doing so won't threaten the patient's well-being. Also, make sure all electrical equipment is inspected regularly and dated.
• See that spilled liquids are wiped up quickly. Never use electrical equipment as a place to set damp towels, trays of food, or other wet items.
• Be especially careful when using electrical equipment around patients with pacemakers, cardiac catheters, or other direct cardiac lines.
• Make sure monitor leads don't touch the side rails.
• When using a defibrillator, make sure *all* dry caked gel is thoroughly scraped off; a fresh application is applied just before use; and avoid using too much gel. Otherwise, electrical burns may result.
• If a woman patient with an intrauterine device (IUD) is to be treated with short-wave or microwave diathermy of the pelvis or abdomen, make sure the IUD is removed first, or surrounding tissues may be damaged by the heat.

Staff stress

Lack of communication can intensify stress in ICU staff. How to minimize staff stress?

• Make sure that all ICU nurses receive adequate orientation and training before working on the unit or before taking on a more responsible position.

• Keep job-related reference books, manuals, and visual aids available to help all staff members stay up-to-date and informed.

• Schedule regular staff meetings and patient care conferences to foster new ideas and allow staff members to air their problems. Basic problems such as inadequate staffing or lack of supplies always cause stress, but the wear and tear this causes can be reduced if the staff has a chance to talk about these and other concerns.

• Put up a bulletin board for the use of doctors, nurses, supervisors, and all staff.

• Make sure hospital policies are clear, concise, and *written*. Knowing what your responsibilities are can make the job a lot easier.

• If you're in a supervisory position, maintain your objectivity and try to provide members of your staff with the support they need.

include him in decision-making and to avoid restraining him whenever possible. Another patient may become totally dependent during illness and may turn to an authority figure (like you) to solve all his problems. You may have to discourage this behavior once the patient's condition improves, but it may be helpful to let him depend on you until then. Also try to be aware of how the patient interacts with family members. Remember, not all visits are beneficial, and destructive relationships can add to the patient's stress. If certain visitors seem to upset your patient, try to find out why and work with other members of the family to remedy the situation.

How the patient's family copes

Don't forget that the family is also forced to cope with the patient's illness. And family members' reactions to the ICU may be even more intense than the patient's response, since they're better able to see the whole unit, the way the staff treats the patients, the continual hustle and bustle, and the vast array of medical hardware. The complexity of this atmosphere can easily make the family feel helpless. While Mrs. Russell cared for Mr. Russell's "cold" without difficulty at home, when he was on a ventilator in the ICU she was frustrated and felt that her caring role had been taken over by machines and professionals. She couldn't help feeling angry when, while her husband was laboring for every breath, she saw the ICU staff joking around at the nurse's station or enjoying a coffee break in the back room.

In some ways, being a survivor is more difficult than being ill or dying, and family members may feel that the patient has gone away and left them behind to pick up the pieces. If relationships were unstable before the patient's illness, the family may feel guilty and even responsible for his illness. The family may have trouble finding time to visit the patient, getting time off from work, or arranging child care during trips to the hospital. They may find taking over the responsibilities around the house—paying bills, mowing the lawn, doing the laundry— a difficult burden. Financial worries may add to this burden. And, of course, there's the stress of seeing someone they love immobilized and hooked up to monitors and machines; and of waiting endlessly to stay just a few moments with someone who may scarcely be aware of their presence.

The family can help

You may think, "I just don't have time to deal with all this on top of everything else. And besides, the family gets in the way." But reconsider: The family can be a help rather than a nuisance. Family members are, after all, your best link with the patient. They know his likes and dislikes and may be especially aware of even slight changes in his condition. While teaching them patient care may be time-consuming, it pays off: The care the family gives can make your job easier; it lets the family feel less helpless and gives the patient at least a small chance to feel closer to those he loves.

Orienting the family to the ICU can help eliminate fear. Monitor the effect of family visits on the patient—perhaps they'll give him the stimulus he needs to strengthen his will to live. Don't forget to relay family messages. And if the family denies the severity of the patient's condition, don't ignore this or misrepresent the situation when the outlook is undeniably bleak. Make sure the family understands the patient's illness and treatment, and keep communications open between all members of the team so the family gets consistent information.

A real pressure cooker

We've been talking about how patients and families respond to the ICU. But how about its effect on the staff? Just what frustrations and sources of satisfaction does the ICU offer? The ICU is a real pressure cooker, with the staff coping constantly with crises. Work in the ICU requires repetitive routines, attention to tiny details, sharp observation, quick and irreversible decisions, and the effective use of highly sophisticated equipment—all in a very limited amount of space, with a virtual obstacle course of cords and wires.

This highly charged environment is filled with highly charged people. The challenge of ICU naturally attracts nurses who are extremely competitive, strong-willed, independent, aggressive, and highly motivated, which may lead to friction among members of the staff. Doctors may not be available at times of critical intervention, or they may not respond to your call for help if they don't agree with your assessment of the situation. The floor where the patient's transferred after leaving the ICU might not continue the patient teaching you began. Patients and their families might be unwilling, or unable, to

Legally speaking

Whenever you practice nursing, but especially in the ICU, follow these guidelines to minimize legal risks:

• Know your equipment. Recognize possible malfunctions—frayed, cracked, or exposed wires; beds that aren't properly grounded; call bells that don't work—and report them to the proper authorities. Always alert the staff, and document what you report.

• Document and report all patient care, and the patient's reaction. Don't just report services rendered to the patient—include everything you see, hear, and feel.

• Note the exact time you make observations, give treatment, or notify the doctor or other personnel.

• When giving assignments, make sure they're within the scope of the person's education and experience. Supervise all personnel under you.

• Before you carry out orders, make sure:

    You're supervised, and that you've had training in the procedure, understand the reason for it, and the effect.

    —The doctor did give the order, or that standing orders or a written policy have been set up by the institution.

• Always maintain patient safety and comfort.

• Continue to grow professionally by attending conferences, classes, or workshops and record the dates and details of all special training you've received. Make sure your employer also keeps such records, and that your work performance is evaluated periodically.

• Obtain special training and a certificate in CPR.

• Buy professional liability insurance.

accept the care you provide, and the patient may be unable to communicate, leaving you to be the only active participant. Later, after the patient improves and can participate, he's transferred to another floor. This is what happened with Mr. Russell. As soon as he could breathe without difficulty, he was taken off the ventilator and transferred.

The ICU has a high mortality rate, but the medical profession is oriented toward preserving life. This paradox leads to a situation in which death is rarely discussed, and in which it's seen as a bitter defeat after the hard struggle to save a life. To put some distance between you and inevitable death, you may be tempted to avoid a patient and his family when there's little hope. Or you may concentrate on technical competence with the sophisticated equipment to give you the feeling you did all that was possible to save a life.

High status
In spite of this strain, the ICU can be a fulfilling place to work and continues to attract highly capable personnel. The opportunities for crisis intervention and decision-making can be very satisfying, and the continually changing variety of patients keeps the work from becoming too repetitive. While tensions may exist among ICU staff members, the high status given the unit, plus the chance to work closely with doctors, can create a sense of camaraderie among team members. And the availability of equipment and supplies in the ICU usually far exceeds that in other parts of the hospital, reinforcing the sense of working in an important, high-priority area. In addition, the very situations that may create stress—giving emotional support to patients and families, using complicated equipment, and facing crisis and death—can all give a sense of meaningful accomplishment when handled well.

While certain stresses in the ICU are inevitable, some of them can be eliminated. For example, rotating patient assignments carefully can give nurses time to teach and work with patients and families. Regular team meetings with a staff psychiatrist, social worker, or psychiatric nurse practitioner can help you cope with patients, their families, and the intensity of the ICU environment. Some have even suggested that "ICU syndrome" can be prevented by giving intensive care nurses the opportunity to rotate. The ICU is truly a special place. With effort and planning you can help make it less stressful.

SKILLCHECK 1

1. Mrs. Tyler is admitted to your unit for shortness of breath and weight gain. List the three basic parts of the nursing assessment you'll make of Mrs. Tyler during your morning rounds.

2. Which of the following definitions correctly describes percussion?
a) Listening to sounds
b) At-a-glance assessment
c) Use of touch
d) Use of tapping to elicit vibrations.

3. Sleep deprivations:
a) Can be avoided by giving large doses of sedatives
b) May be prevented by allowing patients to sleep for 30-minute periods without interruption
c) May cause abnormalities in mental function lasting up to 10 days
d) All the above.

4. Injury and the danger of bodily harm are factors that may directly cause:
a) Psychologic stress
b) Hallucinations
c) Delirium
d) All the above.

5. Ralph Gertner, a 36-year-old auto mechanic, is admitted to your unit for evaluation of abdominal pain. While using percussion on his abdomen as you make your initial assessment, you detect a loud, bell-like, high pitched sound. What might this indicate?
a) Intestinal obstruction
b) Inflammation, as in appendicitis

c) GI bleeding
d) Intestinal gas.

6. In light palpation, you place your entire palm on the patient's abdomen, and:
a) Press down with the heel of your hand
b) Place your other hand on top and press down with both hands
c) Press down with your fingertips
d) Press down with both your palm and your fingers.

7. You're on the committee writing a procedure manual for your hospital's new CCU, and the committee's come to the section on defibrillators. During one of your meetings, a nurse who's recently transferred from another hospital suggests pregelling the defibrillator paddles when there's a chance they may have to be used, since this saves time in an emergency. This has never been done in your hospital, but some of the other nurses on the committee think it sounds like a good idea. What would you add to this discussion?

8. You're working in the ICU, and caring for Mr. Freitas, a COPD patient with pneumonia. Despite his critical condition, Mr. Freitas acts extremely independent. He's constantly trying to get out of bed and sometimes acts hostile and uncooperative. How can you best cope with Mr. Freitas' behavior?
a) Restrain him immediately to protect him
b) Include him in decision-making and avoid restraining him
c) Sedate him
d) Warn him that you'll have to restrain him if this behavior continues.

(Answers on page 183)

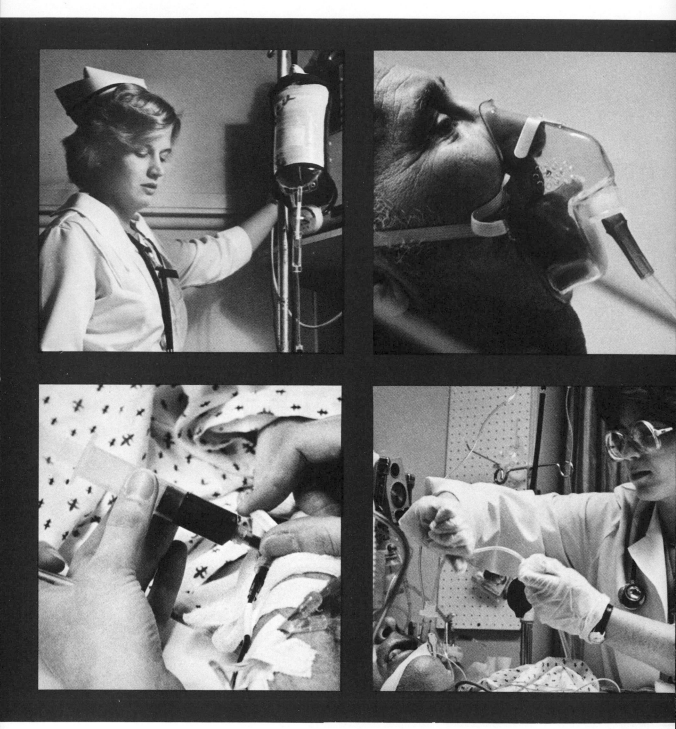

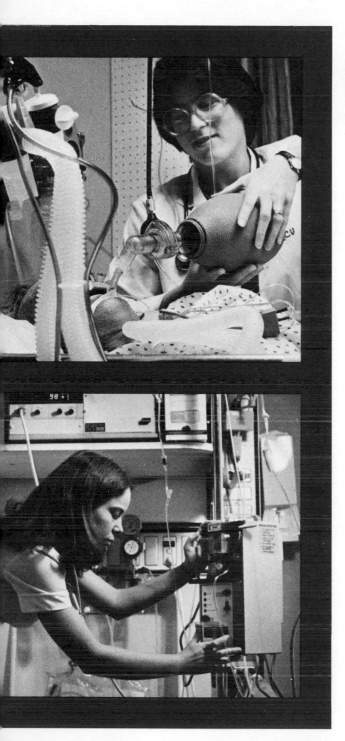

SUPPORTING FALTERING VITAL SYSTEMS

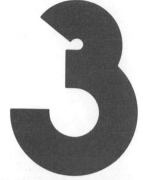

CHRONIC RENAL FAILURE
Compensating for physiologic imbalance

BY CINDY BUTCHER, RN, BSN, HARRY GREENE, MD,
AND PATRICIA DOLAN, RN, BSN, MA

UNLIKE ACUTE KIDNEY FAILURE, which is something the patient usually recovers from, chronic renal failure can follow a downhill course, becoming treatable only by dialysis or an organ transplant. Certain kinds of renal functional impairment (for example, those associated with hypertensive nephrosclerosis and analgesic nephropathy) can be arrested or even improved. But chronic kidney failure can progress from mildly impaired renal function entirely compatible with normal life expectancy, to end-stage kidney failure, and to frank renal insufficiency associated with accumulation of nitrogenous wastes (uremia) and profound physiologic imbalance. In patients with severe renal failure, good nursing care can help prolong life and improve the state of well-being. This chapter will tell you how to give the kind of nursing care that will combat uremia and help relieve its symptoms.

Profound physiologic problems

Chronic kidney failure produces serious metabolic derangements, including glucose intolerance, rising serum triglyceride levels, accumulation of nitrogenous wastes, electrolyte imbalance, anemia, hypotension or hypertension, psychologic

HOW THE KIDNEYS WORK

The kidneys regulate water, blood solutes, and electrolytes; along with the lungs, they also regulate acid-base balance. Through an enzyme called renin the kidneys help control blood pressure, and through a glycoprotein called erythropoietin they stimulate red blood cell formation. They also promote vitamin D metabolism.

The structural and functional unit of the kidneys is the microscopic nephron. There are about 2 to 3 million nephrons in a normal pair of kidneys. Nephrons are wonderfully adaptive—up to 80% of them may be lost before kidney function begins to fail. Those remaining undergo hypertrophy and hyperplasia to maintain function.

A nephron is composed of 2 parts—the corpuscle (a little head) and the sections of the tubule (an endless tail, with a convoluted proximal part and a convoluted distal part separated by a deep U-turn called the loop of Henle).

The length of the nephron's tubules is necessary for increased surface area for absorption and reabsorption.

The glomerulus is a tuft of capillaries in the nephron's head. Set in the cortex, or outer layer of the kidney (an area richly supplied with blood), each tuft branches off one of the many interlobular arteries. The glomerulus is encased in a small sac called Bowman's capsule.

Although it's part of the corpuscle, Bowman's capsule leads into the renal tubule. A protein-free plasma continually passes out of the glomerular capillaries, fills the tiny capsule, and flows along the tubule to receive wastes and furnish materials for reabsorption as the kidney does its chemical work. About 87% of the glomerular filtrate is reabsorbed in the proximal tubule, and the remainder in the loop of Henle, distal tubule, and collecting duct. During this journey the filtrate becomes increasingly concentrated and turns into urine.

The tubules and collecting ducts are finally pulled together into pyramid-shaped masses, which form the middle part of the kidney, or medulla. Each kidney contains 10 to 15 of these pyramids. The pyramid's apex, or papilla, contains the common duct formed from all the collecting ducts of the tubules as they meet, and tapers down to fit into the minor renal calyx, a small, cup-shaped tube. The minor renal calyces open into the major renal calyces in the inner region of the kidney, a hollow collecting chamber called the renal pelvis. This opens into the ureter.

Healthy kidneys are remarkably efficient. Each day they convert 180 liters of plasma into filtrate. Of this, only 1 liter is excreted as urine; the remaining 179 liters are reabsorbed by the tubules and returned to the circulation.

---

disturbances, dermatologic symptoms, and altered reproductive status.

The effect of kidney failure on electrolyte imbalance is particularly pervasive and difficult to correct. Most patients with kidney failure excrete too little sodium. If so, they're vulnerable to ascites. But a few with salt-wasting failure excrete too much. If their urine output is adequate, patients with chronic kidney failure may excrete enough potassium to maintain normal levels until oliguria intervenes. Hyperkalemia is unusual because of certain adaptive mechanisms—including the transcellular movement of potassium into the intracellular space. Kidney failure causes acidosis because excretion of the hydrogen and bicarbonate ion can't keep pace with the acid load. Then, the lungs must excrete more CO_2 (hypocapnia) to maintain some kind of acid-base balance. So, you may notice a change in the patient's rate and depth of respiration. Hyperuricemia, another common finding, can progress to clinical gout, though it rarely does.

Calcium-phosphorus balance also becomes disturbed. The kidneys are unable to appropriately reabsorb phosphorus and calcium. Then, calcium falls in compensatory response to the elevated phosphorus. Patients in chronic kidney failure develop severe bone abnormalities (fractures, calcifications, demineralization, renal osteocysts, and retarded growth in children). Because bone is absorbed and releases calcium in an attempt to maintain a normal serum calcium, these bone abnormalities can be worsened by secondary hyperparathyroidism.

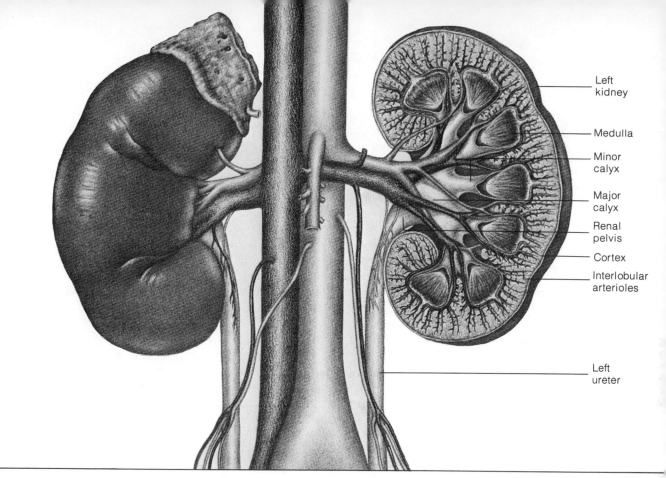

Left
kidney

Medulla

Minor
calyx

Major
calyx

Renal
pelvis

Cortex

Interlobular
arterioles

Left
ureter

Blood and circulatory abnormalities are also common. Anemia results from decreased production of erythropoietin, shortened red-cell survival, and iron utilization; the hematocrit tends to be only ⅓ of normal in kidney failure. Hypertension seems related to fluid retention or disturbance of the renin-angiotensin system which regulates the adrenocortical secretion of aldosterone.

Uremic syndrome
Of course, many of the serious symptoms in patients with kidney failure grow out of the uremia itself. These symptoms may be *gastrointestinal*: anorexia, nausea, vomiting, hiccups, and GI bleeding; *cardiopulmonary*: pericarditis, pleuritis, congestive heart failure, murmurs, pulmonary edema, pleural effusion, and left ventricular hypertrophy; and *CNS abnormalities*: personality change, hallucinations, confusion, irritability, tremors, muscle twitching, neuropathy, labile emotions, short attention span, and inability to concentrate. Cardiovascular disease is the leading cause of death in kidney failure.

What does all this mean in practical terms? It means that patients with kidney failure need dietary restriction and medication to control hypertension and calcium-phosphorus metabolism. They'll be anemic, vulnerable to infection, and lack energy. They'll need hemodialysis when uremic symptoms appear. But even with the benefit of dialysis, they'll have serious physiologic problems you must know how to manage.

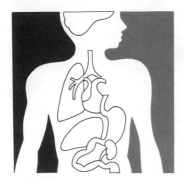

Causes of renal failure
PRERENAL: vascular disorders;
embolism; infarction; CHF;
nephrosclerosis; shock due to
hemorrhage, sepsis, burns,
or cardiogenic shock; placenta
previa; septic abortion; postpartum hemorrhage; eclampsia;
crush injuries; hemolysis; dehydration; surgery in which the
aorta or the renal arteries
are clamped.

INTRARENAL: pyelonephritis,
acute membranous, or membranous glomerulonephritis; Good-
pasture's syndrome; systemic
lupus erythematosus; periarteri-
tis nodosa; scleroderma; diabetes mellitus; amyloidosis;
gout; nephrocalcinosis; heredi-
tary or hypertensive nephropathy; polycystic kidneys; renal
hypoplasia; drugs, heavy metals, or industrial solvents;
acute tubular, or bilateral cortical necrosis; sickle cell disease; radiation nephritis; Wilms'
tumor; hypernephroma.

POSTRENAL: congenital collecting duct anomalies; urethral
strictures; radiation or sansert
fibrosis; pyelolithiasis; carcinoma, lymphoma, or Hodgkin's
disease; prostatic hypertrophy;
urinary tract infection, stones
or obstruction.

Treatment goal

Overall, your goal in caring for a patient in renal failure is to
improve electrolyte balance and combat azotemia by limiting
protein and electrolyte intake. Protein and electrolytes are
controlled largely by diet; fluid level by intake. Much of this
is your responsibility. For example, you'll have to monitor
closely the patient's diet and protein balance. In other words,
you'll help reduce protein breakdown by restricting its intake.
You'll also have to see that the patient gets a high-calorie diet
with supplemental vitamins. Of course, every patient needs
a certain amount of protein as essential amino acids to provide
for tissue repair and maintenance. Otherwise, his body will
metabolize protein from its own tissue and go into negative
nitrogen balance.

Complete proteins containing the best sources of the essential amino acids are eggs, milk, fish, poultry, and meat.
The normal range of protein intake for the healthy person is
from 55 to 60 g per day—about 0.8 g/Kg of body weight. If
allowed 40 g per day, he can have fish, poultry, and meat. But
if he can have only 20 g protein per day, eggs and milk are the
best choices. In any case, every patient needs at least 20 g
protein per day for tissue maintenance, with enough carbohydrates and fat to supply energy and spare the protein for
its own work.

Ordinarily, the dietician assesses the patient's food pref-
erences and plans a regimen just for him. If your hospital has
no dietician, you'll simply have to rely on diet manuals or
nutrition books. Always check the patient's trays to be sure
he is receiving what was ordered. Also, it's a good idea to
record his actual food intake. How many grams of protein is
he actually eating? You'll have to teach the patient and his
family dietary restrictions and their importance.

Other ways to spare protein

Limiting protein intake is not the only way to reduce protein
catabolism. You must also do everything you can to combat
other sources of protein catabolism: tissue necrosis, infection,
immobilization, traumatized cells, internal bleeding, steroids, and fever. What nursing intervention you choose to
accomplish this depends on what shape the patient's in. If he
can get out of bed, encourage him to walk around. If he needs
bedrest, give him careful range-of-motion exercises for all ex-

tremities. Turning a bedridden patient from side to side regularly and caring for his skin will help prevent tissue necrosis.

Remember, too, that special attention needs to be given to the uremic patient's respiratory system. As uremic substances accumulate in the blood, the lungs tend to develop uremic pneumonitis, which may be indistinguishable from pulmonary edema. The cough reflex and respiratory effort are depressed; sputum may be thick and tenacious. Thus, the uremic patient becomes very susceptible to pneumonia. Along with the lessened ventilation that bedrest brings, this makes it especially important to give the uremic patient deep breathing exercises and to use humidified air, IPPB, or good suctioning as needed.

Monitor fluid and electrolyte

Here, your role is critical. You must keep meticulous intake and output records and a daily record of body weight. Remember the rule of thumb: One kilogram of weight gain equals 1 liter of retained fluid. If your patient is alert and able to participate in his own care, let him help decide how to divide his daily allowance of oral fluids; otherwise he may cheat. A leading cause of death in renal failure is congestive heart failure from fluid overload.

One of your most important concerns is for potassium. The crippled kidney can't excrete potassium. Yet, tissue damage, GI bleeding, transfusion, rapid catabolism or sepsis may overload the circulatory system with potassium ions. If diet alone can't control serum potassium, the patient needs more aggressive measures. Hyperkalemia can lead to cardiac arrest. So watch for the characteristic EKG findings in hyperkalemia: high T wave, prolonged P-R interval, absence of P wave, and depressed S-T segment; these may progress to idioventricular rhythm and ventricular fibrillation.

Depending on how urgent his situation is, the hyperkalemic patient may need a calcium infusion to counterbalance the excitatory effect of potassium overload on the heart muscle; sodium bicarbonate, glucose and insulin (to force potassium back into the cells); or polystyrene sodium sulfate (Kayexalate), an ion-exchange resin. This resin works in the gastrointestinal tract to exchange sodium ions for potassium ions, which when bound to the resin, can be excreted. Sorbitol, a substance of high molecular weight, is given with Kayexalate to help excrete potassium by promoting osmotic diarrhea. You

Dialysis differences

In patients in renal failure, either hemodialysis or peritoneal dialysis can be used to remove toxic wastes and excess fluid. But each of these kinds of dialysis has its advantages and disadvantages. Here's a comparison.

PERITONEAL DIALYSIS:
• Can be done immediately.
• Doesn't require complex equipment or highly trained personnel but must be done in a hospital.
• Can't be done soon after abdominal surgery. Takes from 48 to 72 hours.
• Doesn't require the administration of heparin, or requires it only in small amounts.
• May cause more discomfort than hemodialysis.
• May cause peritonitis; shock; atelectasis and pneumonia; severe protein loss; perforation of the bowel, bladder, patent urachus, or blood vessel. In addition, the dialysis fluid may be difficult to retrieve from the abdominal cavity.

HEMODIALYSIS:
• Can't be done immediately, since it requires construction of direct access to the circulation.
• Requires complex, expensive machinery and specialized personnel but may be done in a satellite unit, away from the hospital.
• Requires good blood vessels for the fistula or shunt.
• Takes only 3 to 4 hours.
• Requires the administration of heparin, so there's a risk of hemorrhage.
• May cause septicemia, loss of an artery (or even a limb), embolism, hepatitis, seizures (from rapid fluid and electrolyte changes), and hypotension.

can give Kayexalate by mouth or as a retention enema. The oral route allows the resin to come in contact with more of the GI tract and therefore to pick up more potassium. With 15 g of Kayexalate q.i.d., you can reduce serum potassium by as much as 1 or 2 mEq/L. If you can't, look for hidden sources of potassium. Some medications—penicillins, for example—contain potassium. So do most salt substitutes. Another source to consider—an extracellular shift of K^+ in response to metabolic acidosis. In acidosis the kidneys retain extra K^+ so they can excrete the excess hydrogen ions.

Since sodium retention can cause fluid problems and raise the blood pressure, you'll restrict the patient's dietary intake of sodium. True, Kayexalate is an extra source, but only until it can reduce possibly lethal potassium levels. Besides a low-sodium diet, the patient may need digoxin, diuretics, and antihypertensives to control water retention and hypertension.

Watch for potentially nephrotoxic drugs (aminoglycosides) and drugs that are eliminated or metabolized by the kidneys. If the patient needs such a drug, the doctor should adjust the dose accordingly. Throughout treatment, the patient should have serial renal function tests and monitored serum drug levels. Some drugs that call for such monitoring: amphotericin B, colistin, gentamicin, kanamycin, streptomycin, tetracycline, and digoxin.

Finally, dialysis

If the kidneys continue to fail despite all these measures, dialysis may be necessary. Today, with disposable catheters and commercially manufactured dialyzing solutions, peritoneal dialysis has become a simple and easily accessible method for removing toxic wastes and excess fluid. It's often used to prevent uremia during diagnostic evaluation; while getting the patient in shape for surgery; and in chronic renal failure, especially in patients who lack vascular access or who are hemodynamically unstable. This form of dialysis infuses a solution into the peritoneal cavity through a closed drainage system. It uses the peritoneum as a dialyzing membrane to replace the malfunctioning kidneys. The peritoneum's filtering surface—about 22,000 square centimeters—approximates the surface of the glomerular capillaries. This strong, smooth, colorless, serous membrane lines the walls of the abdominal cavity with its own parietal surface and wraps the abdominal

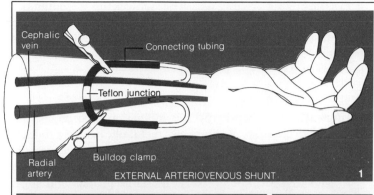

Cephalic vein

Connecting tubing

Teflon junction

Radial artery

Bulldog clamp

EXTERNAL ARTERIOVENOUS SHUNT 1

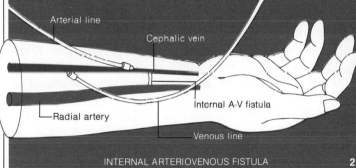

Arterial line

Cephalic vein

Radial artery

Internal A-V fistula

Venous line

INTERNAL ARTERIOVENOUS FISTULA 2

Limited access

Hemodialysis patients must have an access route to deliver their blood to the dialysis machine. There are two ways to provide such access:

1. Provide one external *arteriovenous (AV) shunt*. In an AV shunt, one cannula (tube) is inserted into the radial artery of the forearm and another into an adjacent vein. These cannulas are then brought to the skin surface and are joined to form a continuous circuit. During hemodialysis, blood flows from the arterial cannula through tubing into the machine, and dialyzed blood flows back through the venous cannula.

Teach patients with external shunts to clean them daily. Carefully examine the skin around the shunt for redness, tenderness, drainage, and erosion over the tubing. The tubing should feel warm, and you should feel bruit or thrill. If the tubing is cool, if there's no bruit or thrill, or if you can see blood separation in the tubing, the shunt may be clotted. Report this to a doctor immediately.

External shunts need special attention. Tell the patient to keep the shunt arm wrapped in an Ace bandage at all times to avoid disconnecting the shunt and to avoid injury to or strenuous exercise of the arm. Blood shouldn't be drawn from the shunt arm; nor should it be used for taking blood pressure. Patients should carry a tourniquet and bulldog clamps with them at all times and should know how to use them if the shunt becomes disconnected.

2. *AV fistula* is the preferred access for hemodialysis patients because it's less likely to be damaged or disconnected by trauma, and because it carries a lower risk of infection than the external shunt. In an AV fistula the radial artery is connected to an adjacent vein by a side-to-side, a side-to-end, or an end-to-end anastomosis and is then covered with skin. The vein becomes engorged as arterial blood leaks into the venous system and may readily be punctured for hemodialysis.

To further dilate the vein, the patient applies a tourniquet and exercises the fistula arm before hemodialysis. Using a 14- or 16-gauge needle, the dilated vein is punctured, with the needle pointing toward the fistula. Another needle is placed in the vein, facing away from the fistula, or it may be placed in an adjacent vein. A blood pump on the tubing leading from the first needle to the dialysis machine pulls arterial blood from the vein by way of the fistula. Blood returns through tubing connected to the second needle.

Like a shunt, a fistula should be inspected daily for signs of infection and presence of a bruit or thrill, and the fistula arm shouldn't be used for taking blood pressure or drawing blood. One common problem with a fistula is the "steal syndrome," which is characterized by numbness and ischemia in the access arm. Fistulas may also close up, may lead to aneurysm formation, or may bleed. Patients with such a fistula should know how to apply pressure until bleeding stops.

Three forces in dialysis

1. *Osmosis*: Fluid crossing a membrane moves from a dilute solution to a more concentrated one (as fresh water is drawn into brine). Peritoneal dialysis promotes fluid balance by using a dialyzing solution with a serum-like electrolytic content (except that it ordinarily contains no potassium, because failing kidneys can't excrete it). So you usually add the appropriate amount of potassium with glucose or dextrose to increase tonicity, according to the patient's fluid status. Also, because peritoneal capillaries produce fibrin when irritated, you may need to add heparin to prevent fibrin formation and plugging of the catheter.

2. *Diffusion*: Particles crossing a membrane move from a more concentrated one. In peritoneal dialysis the accumulated waste particles in the blood freely diffuse into the dialyzing bath. Glucose can draw water (and solutes) out of the body, but its molecules are too big to get in readily. So the dialyzing fluid withdraws only small waste particles and water—the amount drawn depends on the amount of glucose put in.

The patient may also need a replacement for ascorbic acid and folic acid lost in dialysis. Once the solution has been infused, it's usually left in the peritoneal cavity for about 20 to 25 minutes. Longer dwell time could result in fluid overload.

3. *Filtration*: Hydrostatic pressure pushes the body fluid out through the body's membranes, then into the abdomen and through the tube, into the collecting bottle below. It depends on the fact that water must seek its own level.

organs inside its visceral one. The peritoneum is continuous in the male, but in the female the ovaries and the fallopian tube jut through it. In peritoneal dialysis the fluid is instilled into the peritoneal cavity between these two layers and is left for a controlled length of time.

Three forces in dialysis

Peritoneal dialysis works by a combination of osmosis, diffusion, and filtration; it drains off metabolic waste products and reestablishes fluid and electrolyte balance. Because the membrane is semipermeable, water and the usual solutes can pass back and forth quite freely; the large protein and sugar molecules much less so. But glucose concentration is not the only factor to influence clearance of the blood in peritoneal dialysis. For example, warming the dialysis fluid enhances solute clearance. Urea clearance is 35% greater at body temperature (37° C. or 98.6° F.) than at room temperature (25° C. or 75° F.). Warming the fluid also decreases discomfort and prevents the patient from losing body heat.

A rapid exchange—finishing the fluid exchange in an hour—increases the efficiency of dialysis. So do volume and concentration. As compared with 1 liter an hour, exchanging 3 liters nearly doubles urea clearance. But for most adults, 2 liters an hour is the least uncomfortable, so this is the standard exchange. Dialysis may start with small exchanges—500 to 1000 ml—and increase by 200 ml per run.

Relative contraindications are those conditions that may decrease the efficiency of peritoneal dialysis: hypertension, collagen disease, vasculitis, lessened peritoneal surface due to infection or surgery (examples: colostomy, a fistula, adhesions or prosthetic materials in the abdomen from previous surgery), recent abdominal surgery, peritonitis, acute abdomen, bowel disease, or ileus. Still, if uremia is life-threatening and hemodialysis is unavailable, peritoneal dialysis is better than nothing, even in patients with these restrictive conditions, *but use with caution*.

In the clearance of certain kinds of waste molecules, peritoneal dialysis is more efficient than hemodialysis. Its greatest advantage, however, is that it can be done in virtually any hospital, without specialist personnel. It can be started quickly, whereas hemodialysis needs special access to the circulation.

In peritoneal dialysis there's usually no need for systemic anticoagulants, with their hazards of hemorrhage. There's a reduced risk of seizures and of hypotension, which are dangerous to patients with coronary or cerebral artery disease, and there is no threat of embolism or of hepatitis.

Some important disadvantages
Peritoneal dialysis is slower than extracorporeal dialysis. It takes from 48 to 72 hours as compared to 3 or 4 hours on a machine. It obliges the patient with a bellyful of fluid to hypoventilate, risking atelectasis and pneumonia. Another serious side effect is the protein loss amounting to 0.2 g to 8 g/liter of dialysate with each exchange—this in someone whose protein intake is already low. Protein deficiency can lead to hypoproteinemia and hypogammaglobulinemia, with ascites, poor wound healing, and perhaps vulnerability to certain infections.

The gravest complication of frequent peritoneal dialysis is peritonitis, a risk that increases with time of dialysis. The infecting organisms are usually gram-negative or staphylococci. Other complications include difficulty in retrieving dialysis fluid from the peritoneum; possible perforation of bowel, bladder, or blood vessel; and shock. Since the female reproductive organs are open to the peritoneum, genitourinary infection could predispose to peritonitis.

Since the dialysis fluid is hypertonic (to promote osmotic diuresis), always consider the possibility of shock, especially if you are using a 4.25% solution. Stay alert for rising pulse rate, which may be the first warning. If blood pressure drops more than 10 mmHg, call the doctor. You may also start oxygen, elevate foot of bed, give medications as ordered, and begin the outflow.

With concentrated solutions, also look out for hypernatremia, hyperglycemia (particularly in the diabetic) and, occasionally, hyperosmolar coma. For these reasons the last exchange should probably be with a 1.5% solution. Also think of air bubbles. Air collects under the diaphragm, stimulating the phrenic nerve, causing a referred pain to the scapular area when the patient is upright. If you suspect an air bubble, put the patient in knee-chest or Trendelenburg position and begin the outflow.

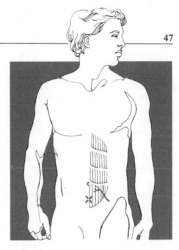

Paracentesis puncture sites
Abdominal paracentesis is the removal of ascitic fluid from the peritoneal cavity. It's done to relieve massive ascites and for diagnostic purposes.

To prepare the patient for paracentesis, have him void to lessen the danger of bladder injury. Place him in a Fowler's position, making sure his back and extremities are supported.

The doctor then chooses a puncture site (see above) and prepares the skin with an antiseptic and a local anesthetic. Through a small incision he inserts a trocar and a cannula into the peritoneum, removes the trocar and connects the cannula to a drainage system. Fluid is drained via gravity for about 15 minutes. This depends on whether the paracentesis is diagnostic or not. Usually the doctor stands by.

During the procedure, reassure the patient. Check his blood pressure, evaluate respiratory status and vital signs often, and watch for signs of hypovolemic shock. Record the kind and amount of fluid removed, which specimen was sent to which lab, and the patient's reaction.

After paracentesis, apply a dressing to the incision.

Dialyzable intoxication

- ALCOHOLS: ethanol, methanol, ethylene glycol
- ANALGESICS: aspirin, methyl salicylate, dextropropoxyphene
- ANTIBIOTICS: cephaloridine, cephalothin, chloramphenicol, isoniazid, kanamycin, neomycin, nitrofurantoin, penicillins, streptomycin, sulfonamides, tetracyclines
- BARBITURATES: amobarbital, barbital, pentobarbital, phenobarbital, secobarbital
- ENDOGENOUS SUBSTANCES: ammonia, bilirubin, lactic acid, uric acid, water
- HALIDES: bromide, fluoride, radioiodine
- METALS: arsenic, Bal-mercury, calcium, potassium, sodium, strontium
- SEDATIVES, STIMULANTS, AND TRANQUILIZERS: amphetamines, dextroamphetamine, diphenylhydantoin, ethinamate, glutethimide, imipramine, meprobamate, paraldehyde, primidone
- MISCELLANEOUS: aniline, boric acid, chlorate, cresol, dichromate, quinidine, thiocyanate

Begin with counseling

Before you bring any peritoneal dialysis equipment to the patient's bedside, the doctor should explain what's involved to both the patient and the patient's family. Be there during the doctor's explanation so you'll know what the patient understands and expects. While you're assembling the equipment and warming the dialysis fluid—warming it to exact body temperature enhances clearance by 35%—you can go over the procedure with the patient according to his understanding of it. Let him ask you questions and talk about his feelings. Later, you can teach him more, as he needs to know it. Include the patient's family in your teaching. They, too, need to understand this long and complex-appearing procedure.

Weigh the patient before dialysis and every 24 hours thereafter, preferably on an in-bed scale. This helps to assess his state of hydration. Also record temperature, pulse, respirations, blood pressure, and central venous pressure (if available) before dialysis.

Dialysis will start to resolve the azotemia, but it's up to you to maintain the strictest sterile technique and to see that the fluid balance and electrolytes swing toward the norm, not away from it. During dialysis keep an exact record of the patient's fluid balance. If less than the amount you infused is returned, record the difference in the cumulative loss or gain column as +, since the peritoneal cavity kept some extra fluid. When you get back more fluid than you infused, mark it as −. At the end of each exchange you'll know what the patient's loss or gain of fluid is. Unless he was retaining fluid to begin with, he should come out about even or slightly negative. Otherwise, he may become seriously overloaded from extended dwell time or inadequate drainage, with consequent congestive heart failure. Keep a record of each exchange, and total it at the end of each shift, including a 24-hour total. Weigh the patient daily (preferably on an in-bed scale), and compare his total body fluid balance to his daily weight record. (Companies that supply your dialyzing solution can also provide easy-to-use forms for maintaining a dialysis record.)

Send a sterile sample of the drainage fluid for culture and sensitivity as frequently as ordered. If the patient has any infection or is HAA (hepatitis-associated-antigen)-positive, consider this fluid contaminated and protect yourself. During the first exchange take blood pressure and pulse every 15 minutes; take them hourly after that. Take the patient's temperature every 4 hours during the exchange and after the abdominal catheter is removed.

Watch for signs of hypernatremia and of hyperglycemia by checking serum glucose and electrolytes. Patients can absorb comparatively large amounts of glucose from the dialysis bath. Check the sugar level closely if the patient has diabetes.

After 48 to 72 hours the sterile dressing and the catheter are usually removed, and dialysis is discontinued. Retaining a catheter for longer than 72 hours sharply increases the risk of infection.

Throughout, one of your most important jobs is respiratory care. Long periods of hypoventilation, enforced by a full abdomen, increase the patient's susceptibility to pneumonia. Raise the head of the patient's bed, and encourage the patient to cough and to breathe deeply often. Turn him from side to side when you can. If he shows marked difficulty in breathing, drain the fluid at once and notify the doctor.

Keep a careful exchange record. If you relieve anyone or anyone relieves you while your patient is being dialyzed—even for lunch break—each one should know the exact status of the exchange and how the recording is to be done. Otherwise there is a risk of making serious errors.

Signs of trouble

Expect the patient to have some pain. The severity of pain varies with the individual. Abdominal pain may be severe at the end of the inflow or outflow periods. This pain can be caused by the dialyzing solution not being at body temperature, by incomplete drainage of solution, or by oncoming peritonitis. If severe pain persists, the doctor will either give 10 ml of 0.5% procaine through the tubing immediately before each infusion, or decrease the volume and give an analgesic. Record it, in any case. If worsening pain is accompanied by rebound tenderness, elevated temperature, or a cloudy effluent, tell the doctor.

Bleeding around the catheter in small amounts is not significant unless it persists. However, it does increase the likelihood of clotting of the peritoneal catheter. Heparin may be given to prevent fibrin formation and plugging of the catheter. Blood-tinged fluid is not uncommon during the first few ex-

Caring for kidney transplant patients

Each year 3,000 Americans receive a transplanted kidney, but over 1,000 of these people lose it to infection or rejection within a year. To avoid these complications stay alert for major signs of rejection: elevated temperature, graft tenderness, decreased urinary output, increased BUN and creatinine, and weight gain. Carefully monitor intake and output, vital signs, daily weight, and state of hydration.

The immunosuppressant drugs given to prevent rejection may make the patient susceptible to infection. To avoid such infection use strict aseptic technique when changing dressings and doing other procedures, and watch for increased temperature or other signs of infection. Wash your hands often, and restrict visitors and staff who have obvious infections. Impose isolation if the patient's WBC falls below 1,000.

Check laboratory results promptly after they're drawn. Immunosuppressants may depress platelet and leukocyte formation, so check these lab values closely. Also, watch for GI ulceration, bleeding, constipation, fecal impaction, and fungal colonization. To reduce the patient's exposure to leukocyte antigens, transfuse only with washed, packed, or frozen red cells.

changes because of subcutaneous bleeding. Normally, the outflow itself is straw-colored.

Cloudy outflow may indicate bacteria. Check its odor. Bloody outflow after the first few exchanges may mean abdominal bleeding. Presence of fecal matter may mean bowel perforation. Copious diarrhea during or after the first exchange may mean bowel perforation; sudden copious urination may suggest bladder perforation. In either case, stop the exchange and notify the physician.

Shock can follow excessive fluid loss. If you see a sudden drop in blood pressure, clamp the drainage tubing and call the doctor.

Protein loss, which is unavoidable, may be significant. Serum albumin determinations should be done daily throughout; an I.V. albumin infusion may be ordered.

Leakage around the catheter calls for frequent dressing change and sterile plastic drapes. Weigh the dressing to estimate the fluid lost (1 g equals 1 ml). Otherwise leave the same sterile dressing in place from beginning to end to cut down on the chance of infection through the incision.

Controlling fluid and dietary intake is an important supplementary way to regulate the burdened kidney. Dietary changes will depend on the changing serum electrolytes and on the creatinine and blood urea nitrogen (BUN) levels. These are determined by blood samples, usually every 6 hours. Also important are continued good care of the skin and range-of-motion exercises.

But with all this, you must make the patient feel that it is he and not the dialysis that is the focal point. Explain everything to him that he wants (or needs) to know. Elicit his help when you can. Make him feel involved and important. And never underestimate the job you're doing: Although it may not take months of specialized training, peritoneal dialysis does need astute, intelligent, and well-organized nursing care to be successful.

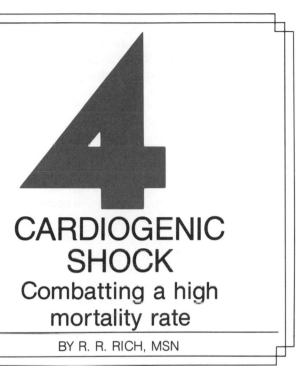

4

CARDIOGENIC SHOCK
Combatting a high mortality rate

BY R. R. RICH, MSN

YOU'RE WORKING IN THE PROGRESSIVE coronary unit (PCU) where several patients are recovering from recent acute myocardial infarctions. You're routinely checking a patient who just yesterday transferred to your unit from the CCU. You find him suddenly much worse and dangerously unstable. He's confused, in severe pain, and his vital signs point to deepening shock. What happened? Your patient developed cardiogenic shock, a perilous complication that strikes many patients during early recovery from acute myocardial infarction. Cardiogenic shock can happen immediately or within 10 days of the infarction. Cardiogenic shock is an important cause of death in patients with acute myocardial infarction. Its mortality rate is generally 80% to 90%—unless vigorous intervention begins immediately!

Do you know exactly how and when to give such lifesaving intervention? Clearly, you must first know how to recognize cardiogenic shock. No less important, you must know how to identify patients in whom this perilous complication is most likely to develop. Cardiogenic shock is sometimes called "pump failure." But it's usually the left ventricle, not the whole heart, which fails. Like other kinds of shock, cardiogenic shock severely impairs oxygen and nutrient transport to the tissues and the removal of metabolites from the tissues. It also causes cardiac output to drop dramatically. To compensate, the body redistributes the available blood supply, shunting blood away from less essential body systems, such as the musculoskeletal and mesenteric, and concentrating it in vital organs, such as the brain and heart. This impaired cardiac function can quickly spell death—unless vigorous intervention begins immediately. Correct intervention aims to improve cardiac function by increasing blood pressure and coronary artery perfusion; improve cardiac output; and preserve ischemic myocardium by decreasing preload, afterload, and myocardial oxygen consumption.

Cardiogenic shock usually develops in patients who have areas of infarction that exceed 40% of the total muscle mass. But certain patients are at greater risk than others. Such vulnerable patients include those who are elderly, have previous infarctions, or suspected extension and those with multiple risk factors including hypertension, obesity, diabetes, smoking or lipid abnormalities. Keeping this high-risk population in mind can help you recognize cardiogenic shock promptly and this is the key to decreasing the high mortality rate. Of course, you must learn to distinguish cardiogenic shock from other kinds of shock. Rule out other possible causes of falling blood pressure and poor cardiac output which characterize cardiogenic shock. These causes include tachyarrhythmias, bradyarrhythmias, hypoxia and drug reactions.

What to look for
The most obvious signs of cardiogenic shock are a precipitous drop in systolic blood pressure; impaired mental function; decreased urinary output; cool, moist, pallid skin; and hypoxemia. Let's look at these telltale signs more closely.

A drop in systolic blood pressure to 30 mmHg below baseline level, or a sustained reading under 90 mmHg that cannot be attributed to medication, often points to cardiogenic shock. Remember, though, in early cardiogenic shock the blood pressure may stay normal at first, as an outpouring of catecholamines attempts to compensate for a weakened myocardium by increasing peripheral resistance and strengthening the force of ventricular contractions. But as catecholamine stores become depleted, and the left ventricle progressively fails, blood

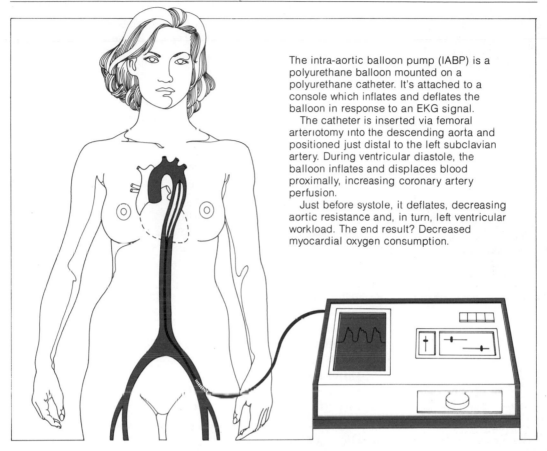

The intra-aortic balloon pump (IABP) is a polyurethane balloon mounted on a polyurethane catheter. It's attached to a console which inflates and deflates the balloon in response to an EKG signal.

The catheter is inserted via femoral arteriotomy into the descending aorta and positioned just distal to the left subclavian artery. During ventricular diastole, the balloon inflates and displaces blood proximally, increasing coronary artery perfusion.

Just before systole, it deflates, decreasing aortic resistance and, in turn, left ventricular workload. The end result? Decreased myocardial oxygen consumption.

pressure falls rapidly and pulse pressure narrows. At first, the patient's peripheral pulse may be rapid and full, as his heart tries to compensate for impending shock, but it soon becomes thready and barely palpable, so be sure to monitor both apical and radial pulses. You can also expect a decrease in urinary output secondary to renal hypoperfusion. Output may fall below 20 ml an hour.

What else should you look for? Because of compensatory peripheral vasoconstriction, the patient's skin is likely to be cool, pale, and clammy, and he may be cyanotic. Cerebral hypoxia may make him apprehensive, restless, or confused, with diminished sensorium and mental alertness. Of course, in a patient who is already critically ill, or who may be receiving narcotics for pain, such mental changes may not be easy to

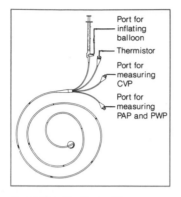

Port for
inflating
balloon

Thermistor

Port for
measuring
CVP

Port for
measuring
PAP and PWP

Securing the Swan-Ganz
The Swan-Ganz thermodilution
catheter is a triple-lumen
catheter inserted into the right
heart to measure cardiac output,
central venous pressure,
pulmonary artery pressure, and
pulmonary wedge pressure.
One port contains a thermistor
tip, to which the cardiac output
monitor is connected.
    The patient who needs Swan-
Ganz monitoring should have
intensive nursing care.
• Before insertion, explain
procedure to the patient. Record
patient's vital signs. Check
position of EKG electrodes and
clarity of oscilloscope signal.
Have lidocaine and a defibrillator handy. Set up equipment
at bedside. Position patient
comfortably, preferably supine,
with his arm extended at an
angle of 60° to 90° to his body
and externally rotated upward.

(continued)

spot. You need accurate baseline admission data and meticulous daily nursing assessments, first in the CCU and later in
the PCU, to detect mental changes that point to cardiogenic
shock.

If an MI patient has all these symptoms—hypotension,
oliguria, altered mental status, and clammy skin or cyanosis—
cardiogenic shock is almost certainly present. But to fill out
the diagnostic picture let's look at Mr. Tracy, whose acute
myocardial infarction of the anterolateral wall was complicated by cardiogenic shock. Mr. Tracy recovered uneventfully
from an inferior wall infarction 3 years ago. But 4 days ago
he was hospitalized again for an acute myocardial infarction.
At admission, his blood pressure was 140/90; apical pulse, 90
and regular; and respiratory rate, 20. He had bibasilar rales
in his lung fields, and his skin was clammy. To relieve his
angina he was given 0.3 mg of sublingual nitroglycerin, and
oxygen at 2 liters, via nasal prongs. He also received prophylactic lidocaine (Xylocaine) 2 mg per minute after a 50-mg
bolus. His vital signs stabilized promptly, and he developed
no cardiac complications. Three days after admission, he was
transferred to the PCU on nitrate therapy and beta blocking
agents.

But 2 days after this transfer, Mr. Tracy became increasingly
confused. His blood pressure dropped to 78/50, his apical pulse
rose to 110, and his radial pulse became weak and thready.
He developed severe chest pain that wasn't relieved by sublingual nitroglycerin and for which he received morphine 7 mg
I.V. Morphine is especially helpful for relieving pain after an
MI, because it produces a beneficial euphoria with fewer cardiovascular effects than most tranquilizers. Morphine also
decreases cardiac workload by arterial dilatation. Such dilatation may be beneficial but could also be dangerous if it
produces systemic hypotension. So keep a close check on
blood pressure in patients receiving morphine. It also can
depress respiratory function—so carefully monitor respirations.

Of course, you have to do more about the MI patient's chest
pain than just give morphine. When an MI patient has chest
pain, take his blood pressure and apical and radial pulses, and
take an EKG (unless otherwise ordered) to help determine if
myocardial ischemia or injury has occurred, or if the patient's
infarction is extending. You may find the S-T segment elevated

or depressed, with the degree of change indicating the amount of myocardial tissue threatened by decreased oxygen supply. The T waves may be inverted, manifesting myocardial ischemia.

Remember, the cardiac patient experiencing angina is severely frightened. Don't add to his fears by showing any hint of panic yourself. When assessing chest pain, always remain calm. Your apparent confidence can help allay the patient's fear, a fear that may intensify his pain. Of course, notify the doctor about every episode of chest pain. In your notes and in your report to the doctor, include the duration, location, quality, and radiation of the pain, any precipitating factors, and the patient's vital signs. If you gave medication for chest pain, record and report the patient's response to it.

Cardiac auscultation during Mr. Tracy's episode of chest pain revealed a new ventricular gallop rhythm—a loud S_3. This low-pitched sound, heard in early diastole, results from a failing left ventricle and has a cadence that sounds like the word "Ken-tuc-ky." At this time, Mr. Tracy's breathing was rapid and labored, and as his pulmonary congestion increased, he began to use the accessory muscles of his thorax to breathe. We could hear moist rales anteriorly at the lung apex. To ease his respirations, we assisted him into a high-Fowler's position and gave oxygen by nasal prongs at 8 liters/minute.

Back to the CCU

Mr. Tracy was clearly in trouble. We connected him to a cardiac monitor and notified his doctor. The monitor can detect the many cardiac arrhythmias that may result from hypoxia and acidosis (common in patients with cardiogenic shock). We prepared for an emergency. We brought a defibrillator, an airway, and an Ambu bag with a face mask into Mr. Tracy's room and placed the floor's emergency cart nearby.

If your floor doesn't have an emergency cart, make sure the following intravenous medications are accessible in case they become necessary: Xylocaine, sodium bicarbonate, epinephrine, calcium chloride, atropine, morphine, and sublingual nitroglycerin.

We assembled an oxygen administration set in the room and continued to assess and evaluate Mr. Tracy's vital signs. Although we'd taken an EKG earlier, we left Mr. Tracy connected to the machine in case we needed another EKG or

Securing the Swan-Ganz
(continued)

If the external jugular approach is to be used, place the patient in Trendelenburg position with towel rolls under his shoulders.
- During insertion, watch oscilloscope for arrhythmias. Monitor and evaluate patient's condition and vital signs.
- After insertion, monitor PAP continuously. Keep the line patent with flush solution. Anchor the transducer to the patient's arm or stationary I.V. pole at RA level.

To flush solution add 500 U of heparin (1:1000 U concentration) to 500 ml bag normal saline solution and label.

Place bag in a pressurized pump bag and inflate to a pressure of 150 mmHg. Maintain this pressure at all times. At this pressure the Intraflow will deliver 3 ml of flush solution per hour.

To inflate the balloon for PCW pressures, proceed slowly until you see a PCW tracing on the oscilloscope. Don't leave the balloon inflated any longer than it takes to record the pressures. Pulmonary infarction can occur when balloons are kept inflated or the PA line is left in the "permanent wedge" position.

Monitoring PA waves
When monitoring patients with a
Swan-Ganz pulmonary artery
line, assess correct catheter
placement by watching the wave
forms on the oscilloscope. For
example, if the catheter inadvertently slips out of the pulmonary
artery into the right ventricle,
you'll see the wave pattern
on the oscilloscope change to
show a characteristic right
ventricular wave pattern. Notify
the doctor immediately so
that the catheter may be repositioned, as ventricular irritability
could result.

Observe pulmonary artery
and pulmonary wedge
pressures to assess patient's
ventricular status and response
to therapy. You'll need to know
the specific wave forms for each
chamber, normal and abnormal
pressures, their significance, and
what they reflect for each chamber (see opposite page).

needed to document a rhythm change. We asked the ward
secretary to call the CCU to find out about bed availability
and to prepare blood requisitions for electrolytes, creatine
phosphokinase with isoenzymes, SGOT, LDH, glucose, BUN,
creatinine, CBC, and arterial blood gases. This expedites the
blood work when the doctor arrives.

The doctor diagnosed Mr. Tracy's condition as cardiogenic
shock, and we prepared him for immediate return to CCU.
The doctor inserted a central line and ordered dopamine (Intropin) started via an infusion pump to maintain a systolic
blood pressure of 100 to 110 mmHg. Dopamine is given through
a central line to avoid infiltration and resulting tissue sloughing
and necrosis. Dopamine is the metabolic precursor of norepinephrine and increases renal and mesenteric blood flow
through selective vasodilation of the vascular beds. It improves
cardiac output through beta stimulation by increasing the force
of contraction. The alpha effect of dopamine produces vasoconstriction.

We called a full nursing report on Mr. Tracy to the CCU,
so the nurses there could prepare for his arrival. During the
transfer to CCU, we monitored Mr. Tracy with a portable
monitor/defibrillator. The airway and the Ambu bag with face
mask accompanied him, along with a portable oxygen tank.

When he arrived in the CCU, the doctor inserted arterial
and pulmonary lines under sterile technique. The nurses made
a baseline nursing assessment. Then they leveled and rebal-
anced the pressure transducer and rechecked the pressure
tubings for the presence of air before recording the initial
intra-arterial pressures. Mr. Tracy's arterial pressure was 80/
64. His pressure would be measured and recorded repeatedly
for regulation of the vasoactive drugs he could receive. Arterial
pressures are usually measured every 10 to 15 minutes until
they're stable; after that, once an hour.

PA line assesses left ventricular function
The doctor inserted a Swan-Ganz pulmonary artery (PA)
catheter at Mr. Tracy's bedside to assess his left ventricular
function. This device is a double or triple lumen catheter that's
inserted intravenously, via a percutaneous approach or venous
cutdown. It's advanced into the right atrium, and the balloon
inflated with 0.8 to 1.5 ml of air. Blood current advances the
balloon catheter. The catheter floats past the tricuspid valve
and through the right ventricle into the pulmonary artery to

P.A. PATTERNS

PA WAVE	PRESSURE INTERPRETATION	NORMAL PRESSURE	SIGNIFICANCE OF INCREASED PRESSURE
Right atrium	Mean right atrial (RA) filling pressure (diastolic) and right ventricular end diastolic pressure (RVEDP).	1 to 6 mmHg	Volume overload; tricuspid stenosis or regurgitation; pulmonary hypertension.

PA WAVE	PRESSURE INTERPRETATION	NORMAL PRESSURE	SIGNIFICANCE OF INCREASED PRESSURE
Right ventricular	Right ventricular pressure (RV).	20 to 30 mmHg systolic, 0 to 5 mmHg diastolic	Mitral stenosis or mitral insufficiency; pulmonary disease; hypoxemia; constrictive pericarditis.

PA WAVE	PRESSURE INTERPRETATION	NORMAL PRESSURE	SIGNIFICANCE OF INCREASED PRESSURE
Pulmonary artery	Venous lung pressure; mean filling pressure of the left atrium (LA), left ventricle (LV), and right ventricle (RV). Pulmonary artery systolic pressure equals RV filling pressure. Pulmonary artery end diastolic pressure reflects left ventricular end diastolic pressure (LVEDP).	20 to 30 mmHg systolic, 8 to 12 mmHg diastolic	Left ventricular failure; atrial septal defect or ventricular septal defect; pulmonary hypertension or stenosis; mitral stenosis.

PA WAVE	PRESSURE INTERPRETATION	NORMAL PRESSURE	SIGNIFICANCE OF INCREASED PRESSURE
Pulmonary wedge	Pulmonary artery end diastolic pressure. Good index of left ventricular heart function.	8 to 12 mmHg	Left ventricular failure; mitral stenosis or insufficiency.

the pulmonary capillary wedge position. Then the balloon is deflated, and the catheter is positioned in the pulmonary artery for pressure measurements. To obtain pulmonary capillary wedge pressures (PCW), the balloon is reinflated and the catheter position confirmed by pressure waveform (see p. 57). In cardiogenic shock, left ventricular compliance is compromised because of depressed cardiac function, so you'll find elevated left ventricular filling pressure.

The PA line also lets you measure the pulmonary capillary wedge, which reflects the left ventricular end diastolic pressure (LVEDP). During diastole, when the mitral valve is open, the LVEDP is transmitted to the pulmonary artery occluded pressure, or PCW pressure.

What's a normal PCW pressure? Usually it's 8 to 12 mmHg, but in cardiogenic shock it may rise above 20 mmHg. This rise in filling pressure during diastole is accompanied by a decrease in cardiac output. One goal of treatment for cardiogenic shock is to reduce the diastolic filling pressure (also called preload). Vasodilators, such as sublingual nitroglycerin, nitroglycerin ointment, or nitroprusside I.V., can accomplish this and are sometimes used together with vasopressors. Vasodilators also decrease systemic vascular resistance (afterload); therefore, direct arterial blood pressure monitoring is a must.

Because of multiple indwelling catheters and invasive procedures, patients with cardiogenic shock are especially vulnerable to infection. Therefore, be sure to maintain strict sterile technique during line insertions and dressing changes. The doctor may order prophylactic antibiotics if insertion procedures are prolonged. In any case, record the patient's temperature every 4 hours unless the patient has a fever; then do it every 2 hours. Draw specimens for CBCs with differentials every 24 hours, and do cultures as needed.

Essential tool

Perhaps the most essential tool for combatting cardiogenic shock is the intra-aortic balloon pump (IABP), a counterpulsation device that increases myocardial oxygen supply, decreases left ventricular work demands, and increases systemic perfusion. The IABP is a balloon catheter inserted via femoral arteriotomy into the descending aorta. It's then positioned distal to the left subclavian artery and proximal to the renal arteries. The balloon catheter is connected to a pumping con-

SOLVING PROBLEMS WITH P.A. LINES		
THE PROBLEM	IF THE CAUSE IS...	THE SOLUTION IS TO...
Damped pressures	Air in system	Check Intraflow, stopcock, and transducer for bubbles.
	Blood on transducer	Flush off or change transducer.
	Clot in system	Aspirate blood until no longer thickened; notify doctor.
	Catheter kinked	Cough patient or extend patient's arm to 90° angle from his body and gently flush catheter. If problem, obtain X-ray.
	Loose connection	Check connections for security.
	Incorrect stopcock position	Correct.
Transducer imbalance	Damaged transducer	Try another transducer.
	Transducer connected to wrong amplifier	Check amplifier connection.
	Broken amplifier	Change it.
Waveform drifting	Insufficient warm-up time	Allow recommended time.
	Cable air vents kinked or coiled	Unkink or decompress.
False low reading	Damped waveform	(See section on damped pressures.)
	Transducer imbalance	Place transducer at heart level.
	Wrong calibration	Recalibrate.
False high reading	Transducer imbalance	Rebalance.
	Flush solution administered too quickly	Pour slow continual flush to 3 to 6 ml/hr.
	Air in system	Remove air from tubing and/or transducer.
Configuration	Improper catheter placement	Try to wedge catheter. Obtain PCW. If problem, obtain X-ray.
	Transducer needs to be calibrated	Recalibrate.
	Transducer not at RA level	Reposition and recalibrate.
	Transducer loosely connected to catheter	Secure.
Drifting wedge pressure (with inflated balloon)	Balloon overinflation	Watch scope while inflating balloon. When waveform changes from a PA to a wedge shape, stop inflating.
PCW pressure trace unobtainable	Incorrect amount of balloon air	Deflate, start again slowly.
	Ruptured balloon	With no resistance to inflation, stop inflation. Notify doctor.

Improve your cardiac and EKG monitoring technique

CARDIAC MONITORING

Readying the patient
• Thoroughly cleanse the patient's skin with alcohol; wipe area dry.
• To insure good skin-electrode contact, you may also apply tincture of benzoin. If the patient's chest is hairy, shave it.
• Make sure all connections between the patient and the monitor fit securely. If the gel pad on the electrode loosens, don't stick it back—replace it.

Selecting leads
• Use a 3- or 5-lead system to monitor the patient. With the 3-lead (3-limb) system, attach the negative electrode directly beneath the right clavicle (RA); the positive electrode on the patient's left chest, below the rib cage (LL); the ground electrode should be placed on the right chest, below the rib cage (RL). This arrangement is Lead II. MCL I (modified chest lead I) is acquired by placing the ground electrode underneath the right clavicle, the negative electrode beneath the left clavicle, and the positive electrode to the right of the sternum 4th intercostal space. With the 5-lead system, the 4 limb leads are placed as follows:
RA is placed beneath the right clavicle
LA is placed beneath the left clavicle
RL is placed below the right rib cage
LL is placed beneath the left rib cage.
• Both these monitoring systems record only one lead at a time. However, you can use the 5-lead system (4 limb leads and chest) to obtain a 12-lead EKG by moving the chest lead to 6 additional positions.
• Connect the electrodes to the

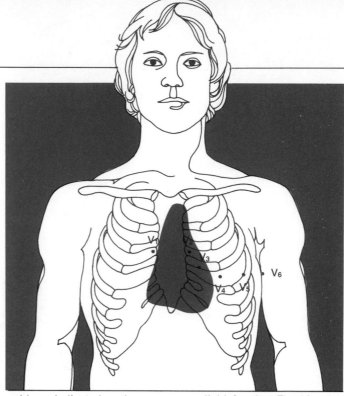

cable as indicated on the cable: right arm (RA), right leg (RL), left arm (LA), left leg (LL). Then attach the cable to the cardiac monitor.

Troubleshooting
• If 60-cycle interference occurs (electrical or mechanical interference that may distort the EKG tracing), try to eliminate it by securing the ground electrode or by tightening loose connections. When this fails, have the hospital medical engineering department check the room for current leakage.
• Set rate alarm parameters close to one another. Rate alarm alerts you of a change in the patient's heart rate. Never turn off an alarm. Use the standby mode only when you are by the patient's side.

EKG MONITORING
Use EKG monitoring for definitive cardiac interpretation, for example, detection of myo-

cardial infarction. The 12-lead EKG helps you look at the heart from all angles, as opposed to the one-sided view afforded by cardiac bedside monitoring.
• Inform the patient of the procedure, and instruct him to relax and stay as still as possible during the procedure.
• Connect the limb leads to the patient's extremities, using alcohol or conductive jelly between the electrodes and the skin.
• Position the electrodes toward the center of the body to minimize artifact produced by strap pulling and twisting.
• While connecting the rubber strap around the extremity, place your thumb on top of the electrode as you pull the rubber strap over your thumb to insure a snug fit. Once the strap is secured, pull your thumb out.

Readying the machine
• Make sure cable-to-electrode connection is secure.

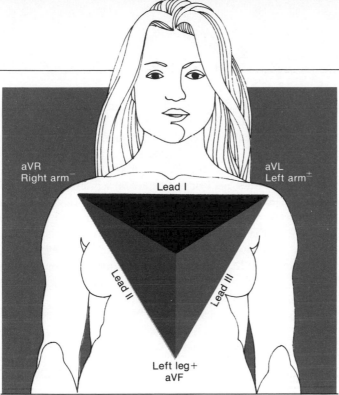

aVR
Right arm⁻

aVL
Left arm⁺

Lead I

Lead II

Lead III

Left leg+
aVF

V₂ at the 4th intercostal space left of the sternum; V₃, midway between V₂ and V₄; V₄ at the 5th intercostal space midclavicular line; V₅ at the 5th intercostal space anterior axillary line; and V₆ at the 5th intercostal space midaxillary line.

• To minimize artifact, apply a sufficient amount of electrode jelly to produce good suction of the cup to the precordial skin, and ask the patient to breathe normally.

• Connect the chest cable to the suction cup, and place it on the chest at the V₁ position. Run a 3-second strip. Proceed through V₆ consecutively, using the markings described above.

• Because the stylus will fluctuate with respirations, it may be necessary to adjust it as the chest leads are recorded.

• When stopping the EKG machine to change the position of the V electrode, be sure to turn the lead selector dial between the V position and CF. If the lead selector dial is turned between V and aVF, "7 aVF syndrome" may occur. This occurs when chest leads are inadvertently recorded using aVF instead of V.

• After completing V₆, run a long rhythm strip on Lead II. Standardize again.

Cleaning up after the test
• Disconnect patient from the equipment, and remove all electrode jelly from the patient with a damp cloth.

• Write the patient's name and the date, time, and room number on the EKG.

• Clean the suction cup of any excess electrode jelly.

• Restock the EKG machine with jelly, paper, and alcohol swabs.

• Loosely coil the cables on the machine to prevent cord and wire damage.

• Check the machine for paper.
• Turn the power on and position the stylus in the center of the paper.
• Turn the lead selector dial to standardization. Set the standardization knob on 1, with paper speed at 25 mm/second. Turn power dial to run, and push the standardization button four times in rapid succession. The standardization marks should be 10 mm high (2 large blocks) when standardization is set at 1. Whenever the half or double standardization is used, make a notation on the EKG tracing.

Recording EKG patterns
• Turn the lead selector dial to Lead I and run a 3-second strip. Mark the leads by depressing the mark button as follows:

Lead	Dash
I	1 short
II	2 short
III	3 short
aVR	4 short
aVL	5 short
aVF	6 short
V₁	1 long, 1 short
V₂	1 long, 2 short
V₃	1 long, 3 short
V₄	1 long, 4 short
V₅	1 long, 5 short
V₆	1 long, 6 short

Continue in this manner from Lead I through Lead aVF, allowing 3 seconds per lead.

After completing aVF, stop the lead selector dial halfway between aVF and the V. Mark the chest positions V₁ through V₆ with a marking pen. This will avoid misleading results and will insure that future EKGs will be taken in the same position. Mark the chest as follows: Using the angle of Louis as a landmark, locate the second intercostal space directly to the right of the angle. Counting down 2 intercostal spaces, locate the 4th intercostal space at the right sternal border. This is the location of V₁. Locate

Places, everyone!

To avoid a chaotic mob scene during a code, try using a team concept. Here are some guidelines. Just one person, usually a doctor or a resident, should give orders and make decisions. Who else should be on hand? An anesthesiologist and inhalation therapist to help maintain ventilation; a pharmacist (present or readily available) to dispense more drugs; a nurse (or two at most) to assist with treatment and record the treatment and the drugs given; and a unit clerk (on standby via the intercom) to call for more personnel or supplies if they're needed. More people than this just cause more confusion.

If your institution doesn't have a written policy on handling a code, or on who should be present, see if one can be developed. It not only prevents confusion—it also improves patient care and uses the available staff more efficiently.

sole, which inflates and deflates the catheter in response to an EKG signal that triggers the pumping action. How does it work? For precise synchronization to the cardiac cycle, an arterial line is required. Optimal timing cannot be done with the EKG alone.

When the balloon catheter inflates during early diastole, it partially obstructs the descending aorta, which displaces blood proximally and distally to increase perfusion of the coronary arteries, systemic circulation, and vital organs. Rapid deflation (just before the next systole) reduces aortic resistance and afterload, thereby decreasing the workload of the left ventricle. Always keep the IABP console set to "auto" (automatic alarm) whenever you're not physically present in the patient's room, because the "manual" setting bypasses the alarm.

The IABP is a remarkable device but carries some additional risks for the patient. The internal presence of the balloon catheter itself necessitates the use of antibiotics. Multiple invasive lines (arterial, PA, IABP catheter) increase the patient's risk of infection. The balloon catheter also increases the risk of thrombus formation and requires full heparinization. Administering the heparin via an infusion pump can reduce the risk of overheparinization. Nevertheless, observe carefully for signs of bleeding and guaiac-test all bodily excreta.

Another important disadvantage of IABP: The mechanical action of the balloon destroys platelets. Closely monitor platelet, hematocrit, and clotting determinations. Clotting determinations are drawn every 12 hours. Make sure the patient's typed and crossmatched for 2 units of deglyceride red blood cells until 24 hours after the balloon has been removed. (Since aortic dissection during IABP insertion is a risk, albeit rare, it's a good idea to have 2 units of blood on hold even before insertion.) Also before insertion, evaluate the patient's bilateral pedal pulses. With an indelible ink marker, mark an X over the area where you feel the patient's pedal pulses. Transient arterial spasms and peripheral embolization may decrease pedal pulses, making them hard to find. Yet, you must monitor peripheral pulses carefully, because inadequate perfusion of the leg may necessitate balloon removal. When monitoring peripheral pulses, also check the color, sensation, and motor function of the patient's leg.

Hip flexion may crack the balloon catheter, reducing IABP efficiency. To help prevent this, frequently remind the patient to keep his "ballooned" leg straight. Avoid raising the patient's head more than 30°; otherwise, elevated positions may force the balloon to move proximally to the aortic notch. Keeping these limitations in mind, be sure to turn these patients regularly. Frequent turning helps reduce the risk of pulmonary complications while maintaining skin integrity. To keep the monitor reliable, always make sure the EKG connections are protected, since IABP dynamics depend on EKG synchronization. Electrode care can't be overemphasized, particularly when a patient is balloon-dependent.

Stability at last

Patients on the IABP should attain hemodynamic stability. Recognize such stability when mean arterial pressure rises to 70 mmHg or greater; PCW pressure decreases to 12 to 15 mmHg; cardiac index is greater than 2 liters; pulmonary congestion decreases; and mental status, urine output, and peripheral perfusion all improve. After the patient maintains such stability for a few days and his overall condition improves, you can begin to wean the patient from the balloon. To do this, the doctor will order the gradual decrease of balloon inflation ratio. The ratio is decreased from 1:1 to 1:2, to 1:4, and finally to 1:8. When the patient can tolerate this last ratio without ill effect, the doctor can remove the IABP in the patient's room, using sterile technique.

Unfortunately, some patients become balloon-dependent—their mean arterial pressure remains under 60 mmHg, PCW persists above 20 mmHg; cardiac index is less than 2 liters; or myocardial ischemia occurs when the ratio of balloon pumping is decreased. The patient may need hemodynamic support—such as vasopressors, vasodilators, or diuretics—during the weaning process. Of course, if the patient develops recurrent chest pain or EKG changes, notify the doctor promptly so he can order reversion to the weaning plateau.

After weaning

During the period after IABP removal, you'll need to work closely with the patient's doctor. He should define an acceptable range for blood pressure, PCW pressure, and urine output, and should leave standing orders for initiating diuretics, nitrates, volume expanders, or vasopressors if the patient deviates from this range. Of course, as always, report recurrent chest pain or EKG changes to the doctor immediately.

We were able to wean Mr. Tracy from the IABP after 3 days. Two days later he was again ready for transfer to the PCU, where the remainder of his recovery was uneventful. At the end of 21 days, he was discharged in good condition, controlled on medication.

While clinical investigation continues in an effort to decrease cardiovascular diseases, the key to decreasing mortality from cardiogenic shock is still early recognition and treatment. Your prompt nursing assessment and correct intervention can play a vital role.

5

RESPIRATORY FAILURE
Monitoring mechanical ventilation

BY HANNELORE M. SWEETWOOD, RN, CCRN, BS

MAINTAIN ADEQUATE RESPIRATION! Nothing you can do for any patient, especially one who is critically ill, can be more important than this. For without the adequate gas exchange that effective respirations provide, all other systems quickly fail.

In patients who are critically ill, promoting adequate respiration is a special responsibility. Studies have shown that most patients in intensive care units have abnormal blood-gas levels. These patients need special respiratory support, often with mechanical ventilation.

The ventilators of today have come a long way from the primitive iron lungs of the 1930s and it takes real know-how to operate them effectively. If you have it, you can competently manage patients with respiratory failure by...

• recognizing the need for mechanical ventilation or other respiratory support

• knowing how and when to begin ventilator therapy; and how to assess clinical response to it

• knowing how and when to wean the patient from the ventilator. This chapter will give you the information you need.

Acute respiratory failure brings a degree of oxygen deficit

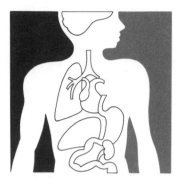

Causes of respiratory failure
AIRWAY OBSTRUCTION:
foreign body aspiration
(vomitus, trauma); inflammation
(epiglottiditis, laryngitis,
asthma, croup); airway burns
(heat or chemicals); chronic obstructive lung disease (COLD);
fibrocystic disease; pulmonary
edema; drowning or near-
drowning.

THORACIC RESTRICTION OR
TRAUMA: flail chest; multiple rib
fractures, penetrating chest
wounds, ruptured diaphragm,
pneumothorax; abdominal
surgery; ascites; peritonitis;
severe obesity; kyphoscoliosis;
spinal arthritis.

NEUROMUSCULAR DEFICITS:
CNS depression (drugs, trauma,
CVA, uncontrolled O_2 therapy);
coma (diabetic, uremic);
disease (Guillain-Barré, polio,
multiple sclerosis, myasthenia
gravis); myoneural junction
involvement (toxins: botulism,
tetanus, organophosphates).

PARENCHYMAL DISEASE:
traumatic pulmonary contusion,
"shock lung" (ARDS);
tumors (benign or malignant).

DISTURBANCES OF PULMONARY
PERFUSION: emboli, fat emboli, or
pulmonary hypertension.

that can rapidly lead to brain damage. So begin to think of hypoxia when you see its characteristic clues: anxiety, confusion, and agitation. The patient may become combative or belligerent (like Mr. Carter, whom we'll describe later on). He'll be extremely short of breath and may or may not be cyanotic. Without oxygen, such a patient will go into acidosis and shock—and may die. So, check the anxious and confused patient at once for a rise in blood pressure and pulse rate. Give him oxygen immediately, in concentrations up to 100%, and have resuscitation equipment, including an Ambu bag, handy. Get someone qualified to intubate the patient, and set up a ventilator ready for use; intubation and ventilation are usually needed. Arterial blood-gas analysis will quickly show the patient's respiratory status and can guide therapy.

Mr. Carter, a 55-year-old plumber, was brought to the emergency room with severe shortness of breath. He was agitated, seemed confused, swore at us, and refused to supply a social and medical history. We noted at once that he was barrel-chested, with very noticeable neck veins in the upright position.

Mr. Carter's test results, combined with his physical appearance, indicated a patient with chronic obstructive lung disease (COLD) reaching an acute stage. Yet why was a man who was actually struggling for each breath using his meager air reserve to fight us off?

Confusion, anxiety, and belligerence are frequently a sign of cerebral anoxia. Never dismiss such a patient's behavior as merely uncooperative or hysterical; he is in real trouble. As hypercarbia mounts, producing CO_2 narcosis, belligerence may be succeeded by more sinister signs—lethargy, disorientation, and stupor. Many patients with Mr. Carter's $PaCO_2$ (68 mmHg) would have been unconscious long before.

If we hadn't thought carefully about all of Mr. Carter's symptoms, we might have inappropriately sedated this raving man, finishing off whatever breathing reflexes he had left. Another respiratory clue: Check to see if the patient is comfortable in a supine position. Notice if he can talk with you normally. He could have orthopnea, the inability to breathe while lying flat. He may also be unable to say more than a few words without pausing for breath. This condition is usually due to incipient pulmonary edema or some other serious respiratory problem.

UNDERSTANDING ABGs

	Normal	Respiratory acidosis	Respiratory alkalosis	Metabolic acidosis	Metabolic alkalosis
POSSIBLE CAUSES		Impaired alveolar ventilation, respiratory depressants, intracranial tumors	Ventilatory support, hyperventilation, CNS disease, anxiety, persistent fever, liver disease, CHF, pulmonary embolism	Aspirin, renal disease, diabetes, lactic acidosis, diarrhea, biliary fistulae	Vomiting, diuretics, hyperadrenocorticism, alkali ingestion, hyperaldosteronism, nasogastric suction
SYMPTOMS		Lethargy, shallow irregular respirations, disorientation	Hyperactive reflexes, blurred vision, tetany, vertigo, muscle cramps, sighing, diaphoresis	Kussmaul's respiration, restlessness, disorientation	Weakness, paralysis, leg cramps, paresthesias
SIGNS		Hypoventilation, asterixis	Hyperventilation, latent tetany	Shock, coma, tachypnea, almond odor from mouth	Hypokalemic symptoms (nausea, weakness)
pH	7.35 to 7.45	Normal or decreased	Increased	Decreased	Increased
PO_2	90 to 95 mm Hg	Decreased	Altered	Normal or increased	Normal or decreased
PCO_2	34 to 46 mm Hg	Increased	Decreased	Decreased	Increased
HCO_3	24 to 26 mEq/L	Increased	Decreased	Decreased	Increased
RR*	10 to 20/min.	Irregular	Altered	Increased	Decreased

*Respiratory rate

COMMON METHODS OF OXYGEN ADMINISTRATION

EQUIPMENT	LITER FLOW	O₂ CONCENTRATION	HUMIDIFICATION	TYPE OF PATIENT
Nasal cannula	2 LPM	About 24%	Bubble humidifier	Chronic obstructive pulmonary disease (COPD)
Nasal cannula	7 LPM	About 35%	Bubble humidifier	Most cardiac patients
Venturi mask	4 LPM (follow manufacturer's instructions)	24%, 28% etc. (marked on mask)	Bubble humidifier sometimes with special fittings for high humidification	Chronic obstructive pulmonary disease (COPD)
Aerosol mask	8 LPM	40%, 70%, 100% depending on setting*	High-humidity humidifier such as Puritan or Ohio Nebulizer	Most respiratory infections following extubation
High concentration nonrebreathing mask	10 to 15 LPM	95%	Bubble humidifier	Severe pulmonary edema, pulmonary embolism, or other conditions of severe hypoxia

*The amount of O₂ actually delivered to the patient is less than indicated by the setting, and varies with rate and volume of respirations. Regulate dosage according to the patient's needs.

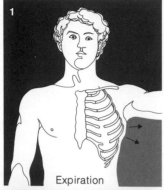

Expiration

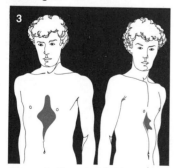

Inspiration

Figures 1 and 2: *Flail chest.*
Paradoxical motion of the chest
wall during breathing due to
multiple rib fractures or disrup-
tion of several costosternal
cartilages.

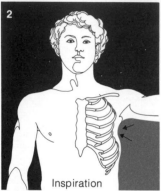

Figure 3: *Funnel chest* (pectus
excavatum). Marked depression
of the sternum, probably due
to a congenital deformity.

Next examine the vital signs. Mr. Carter's vital signs were:
respirations, 30 and labored, with some rales and wheezes
on auscultation; pulse, 115 and slightly irregular; BP, 180/95;
ABGs: $PaO^2 - 55$ mmHg and $PaCO_2 - 68$ mmHg; and pH 7.25.

Recognize a respiratory rate in a resting adult below 12
and above 25 as a trouble signal. Mr. Carter's rate was a
danger-alerting 30. But keep in mind that an adequate respiratory rate alone does not guarantee adequate lung ventilation. The depth of respirations is equally important. We
assessed Mr. Carter by observing the excursions of his diaphragm and thorax, and by listening for his breath sounds
with a stethoscope.

Do not mistake rapid, shallow respirations for hyperventilation; they do not provide adequate oxygenation and CO_2
removal. Mr. Carter's labored breathing was another red alert.
Use of auxiliary respiratory muscles during rest or mild exercise is always a sign of respiratory distress.

Observe the chest for equal expansion. Decreased movement of one side may be due to pain or an underlying problem
such as fractured rib(s) or pneumothorax. In accident victims,
watch for flail chest (see insert).

Check the position of the trachea. A deviation from the
midline may be due to tension pneumothorax, an immediately
life-threatening condition. Be aware that musculoskeletal deformities, such as Mr. Carter's barrel chest, may indicate pulmonary disease (see insert). And that obese patients have an
added risk of respiratory complications.

Cyanosis: A late sign

Remember that dangerous hypoxia may exist long before cyanosis becomes visible. Expect to see cyanosis first in the
buccal membranes. If hypoxia is chronic it may produce clubbed
fingers and toes, a visual clue that's common in Fallot's te-
tralogy and chronic obstructive pulmonary disease.

Patients with acute pulmonary disease such as pulmonary
embolism, or chronic disease such as emphysema, may develop cor pulmonale—right ventricular heart failure. Review
them for signs of this ailment: distended neck veins that persist
when the head is elevated above a 45° angle, a tender, enlarged
liver, and dependent edema, aching abdominal pain, and increased venous pressure. Such patients usually show a positive
hepatojugular reflex.

Establish an airway

Once you have recognized respiratory distress, your first step is to establish a patent airway. Position the head of any obtunded or comatose patient so his tongue can't fall backward occluding his airway. Be sure to inspect the patient's mouth carefully. Remove loose dentures, blood, vomitus, and other foreign materials. Use an oral or nasal airway to keep the tongue in the correct place and facilitate suctioning.

Teach cooperative patients to improve their own ventilation with proper breathing technique. To prevent complications in postoperative and bedridden patients, encourage them to take several deep breaths every hour while awake. Teach them to use the diaphragm while inhaling by pulling in the stomach during exhalation. This will cause automatic use of the diaphragm on the next inspiration. Teach patients with chronic pulmonary disease to inhale and exhale to the count of four. This will produce smooth, even ventilation of the lungs, helping to prevent respiratory panic during acute asthma attacks or exacerbation of chronic obstructive lung disease (COLD). Help the patient to an upright position for his breathing exercises. If he's bedridden, turn him frequently; if not, make sure he's walking some time each day. Both turning and walking improve ventilation.

When to ventilate?

Whenever the patient's own respiration can't maintain adequate pulmonary gas exchange, some kind of respiratory support is needed. When hypoxemia can't be corrected, even with high concentrations of supplementary oxygen, mechanical ventilation should begin. To know when this is so, you must evaluate the state of oxygenation (PO_2) and adequacy of CO_2 elimination (arterial PCO_2.) But more important than the absolute numbers shown in the PO_2 and PCO_2 result is the patient's condition. There's no absolute PCO_2 level at which intubation and mechanical ventilation are *always* indicated. But decompensated respiratory failure with respiratory acidosis (low arterial pH) leading to obtundation not reversible by conservative measures, means mechanical ventilation should begin.

You know it's time for mechanical ventilation when respiratory distress changes to respiratory failure, leaving the patient unable to maintain adequate oxygenation (hypoxemia)

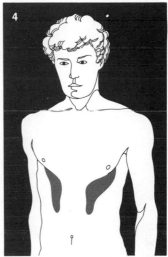

Figure 4: *Pigeon chest* (pectus carinatum). Undue prominence of the mid or lower sternum due to congenital deformity.

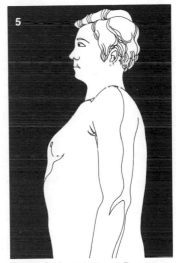

Figure 5: *Barrel chest*. Round bulging chest with an increase in the anterior, posterior diameter of the chest; usually the result of chronic air trapping in the lungs or hyperinflation of the lungs. Seen in emphysema.

and/or carbon dioxide removal (hypercarbia) without straining to breathe. Generally, respiratory failure is described as a PO_2 below 60 mmHg, a PCO_2 above 49 mmHg, or both. The ventilator, as it's often more appropriately called, breathes for the patient.

If the patient needs a ventilator, you must establish an effective airway. Get someone to place an endotracheal tube if the patient is unconscious or if you expect a short-term need for ventilator therapy, as in drug overdose. If intubation is impossible because of trauma, the patient will need a tracheostomy.

Pressure or volume ventilators

To use ventilators effectively, you should know the essential differences between the two kinds:

Pressure ventilators are driven by gas (air or oxygen) and deliver gas into the patient's airway until they produce a preset pressure. These ventilators (examples, Bird Mark 10, Bennett PR II) are not generally used for long-term mechanical ventilation. They're useful in emergencies because they're portable; but their major use is for IPPB treatments.

Generally, IPPB treatments are used to administer oxygen; to administer aerosol medications; to expand the lungs; and to facilitate removal of secretions. They're usually given by a respiratory therapist. Your responsibilities to patients receiving IPPB treatments include the following:

• Monitor pulse and blood pressure carefully, especially if the patient is receiving sympathomimetic medications (for example, Isuprel).

• Assess response to treatment.

• Watch for complications or side effects.

• Provide information, instruction, and reassurance, as needed.

Volume ventilators are electrically powered and deliver a preset tidal volume whenever the ventilator is triggered. Then a piston or bellows pushes a predetermined volume into the patient's lungs at a fixed rate. You can vary inspired oxygen concentrations between 21% and 100% by changing the oxygen flow to the ventilator. Volume ventilators are less affected by changes in pulmonary mechanics. They are the kind generally used for continuous mechanical ventilation.

Although respiratory therapists are usually responsible for

the functioning of ventilators, you should know basically how they work so you can respond effectively to alarms and provide appropriate patient care. The major controls on volume ventilators (Bennett Ma-1) are these...

• *Tidal volume control* determines the amount of air delivered to the patient with each inspiration.

• *Respiratory rate control* determines the number of breaths per minute. When the patient himself initiates respirations (assisted ventilation), this is set at a rate lower than the patient's own, so the ventilator will take over automatically if the patient's respirations slow down or stop altogether.

• *Pressure limit control* determines the maximum amount of pressure to be created in the patient's airway. If the pressure created exceeds this limit, the remainder of air will escape through a safety valve. This sets off an audible alarm and lights up the pressure indicator. Check the patient when this happens. It's usually a sign that he needs suctioning.

• *Oxygen dial* controls selection of concentrations from 21% (room air) to 100%. If the ventilator can't deliver the preset oxygen concentration, an alarm sounds and the indicator light turns red.

• *Sensitivity control* determines the inspiratory effort the patient must make to trigger the respirator. This control is usually shut off when IMV or PEEP are in use.

Monitoring ventilators

To insure effective use of ventilators, check inspiratory pressure, ventilator rate, and expired tidal volume hourly. Check results against doctor's respiratory orders. What if the results of your hourly check are not on target?

• Look for leaks at connection sites—humidifier, tracheostomy or endotracheal cuff, exhalation balloon or cuff.

• Look for air flow obstruction—large accumulations of secretions or mucous plugs in the endotracheal or tracheostomy tube, or in the airway. If you find such obstruction, suction thoroughly.

• When using a pressure-limited ventilator, to avoid oxygen toxicity in patients who need long-term ventilation, use compressed air for your pressure source. Then, bleed in sufficient oxygen to keep arterial oxygen tension within normal range.

• Keep the alarm in the "on" and "continuous" positions.

• Periodically check the tidal volume, rate, and FIO_2 (frac-

The sounds of breath

HEARD WITH UNAIDED EAR:
• *Stridor* sounds (croupy, hoarse, metallic) are caused by upper airway obstruction.
• *Grunting* sounds are caused by airway obstruction or by a neurologic reflex in head-injury patients.

HEARD WITH STETHOSCOPE:
• *Bronchial* sounds (loud, high-pitched, with a distinct pause between inhalation and exhalation) are normal over the trachea or bronchi; abnormal over other lung areas. Abnormal bronchial sounds (tubular) indicate consolidation of pulmonary tissue.
• *Vesicular* sounds (soft, low-pitched, with a rustling quality and no pause between inhalation and exhalation) are normal over lung areas other than trachea or bronchi.
• *Absent or diminished* sounds may indicate many abnormalities, such as an obstructed airway, pneumothorax, or pleural effusion.
• *Fine, crepitant* (popping) rales heard over the dependent portion of the lungs are due to air movement through fluid in the alveoli.
• *Moist, coarse* (loud, low-pitched gurgling) rales occur when excessive secretions move through the bronchioles.
• *Friction rub* (leathery, rubbing sounds) may indicate pleural disease and may be heard in pulmonary infarction.
• *Egophony* is an abnormal sound heard in pleural effusion: When the patient says the letter "e", its sound changes to "a."
• *Whispered pectoriloquy* is another abnormal sound heard over areas of pleural effusion. As a patient whispers, you can distinguish words over the areas of effusion or consolidation, not over areas of normal lungs.

Treating the tracheostomy

- Treat the tracheostomy site as a surgical wound. Use sterile technique, wear gloves, and wash your hands before and after suctioning.
- Suction as needed but only during withdrawal of the catheter and only 5 to 10 seconds at a time.
- Allow the patient to breathe, or ventilate him with a ventilator, after each passage of the catheter.
- Ventilate the patient with 100% oxygen before, during, and after each suctioning.
- Avoid too vigorous suctioning, which could cause severe tracheal injury.
- Change the sterile humidifier and nebulizer every 24 hours; change sterile water and tubing every 8 hours.
- Discard water condensed in tubing as necessary.
- Change dressing (sterile precut gauze) every 8 hours.
- Routinely culture tracheal aspirate at least every 3 days. Check and record color change, consistency, and amount of secretions.
- Inspect the site frequently for bleeding, hematoma formation, and for possible dissection of air through the tissue of the neck.
- When the patient is to begin oral feeding, offer water first to make sure he can swallow without aspirating.
- Deflate the cuff only if a significant change occurs in the airway pressure.

tional concentration of inspired oxygen) dials to see that they haven't been moved from the prescribed settings.

- Keep a log of intentional setting changes for each dial taped to the machine along with a flow-sheet showing arterial blood-gas readings, ventilator settings, and vital signs.
- Keep the humidifier filled with sterile, distilled water to the level marked. To see that it's working correctly, make sure it's never cold and watch the delivery tubings. They should always contain some moisture. But if you see actual water accumulation, empty it, at least once an hour. Water might obstruct the flow, and contaminate and flood the trachea.
- IMV (intermittent mandatory ventilation) may be used to exercise the respiratory muscles of the patient who can maintain spontaneous inspirations.
- Coordinate the drawing of arterial blood gases with changes in ventilator settings. Whenever you change the ventilator setting, remember to wait 20 minutes before drawing the next sample. This allows the patient time to respond to it.

What complications?

Any patient who needs positive-pressure mechanical ventilation needs endotracheal or tracheostomy intubation. Once thus intubated, he's no longer able to warm and humidify the inspired gas, or keep his airway sterile. Such a patient is vulnerable to atelectasis and pneumonia, since lack of humidification promotes drying and retention of secretions. Retained secretions can obstruct airways and lead to infection. So, the mechanical ventilator should have a heated humidifier capable of delivering gas saturated with water at approximately body temperature. Another problem is potential contamination from bacterial growth in the ventilator equipment itself.

Clearly, the ventilator patient requires special care. Weigh him daily—a positive water balance with resultant interstitial pulmonary edema is often a side effect of mechanical respiration. Keep track of the patient's nutritional status and monitor his fluid intake and output. Make sure adequate nutrition is provided by tube, hyperalimentation, or oral feedings. Also, carefully monitor blood gases for adequate oxygen/CO_2 exchange. Keep infections to a minimum by using strict aseptic technique. Watch for mucous plugging, common in dehydrated patients. Regularly auscultate all lung fields to check endotracheal tube placement. A misplaced tube could cause lung

HOW TO DO POSTURAL DRAINAGE EXERCISES — PATIENT TEACHING AID

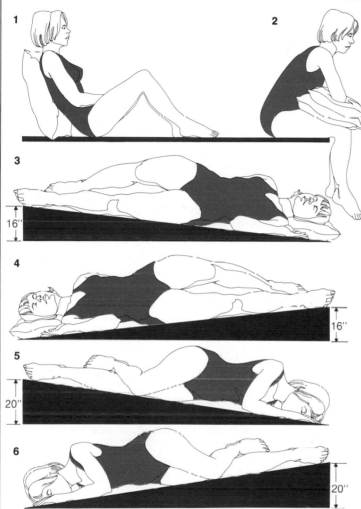

higher than your head. Lie on your left side, with a small pillow under your head and pillows behind your back. Lean back slightly on the pillows. Have someone clap or vibrate the front of your chest over the nipple and just below it on the right side.

4. Position yourself as you did for Exercise 3, but this time turn to your right side. Have someone clap the left side of your chest.

5. Include this important exercise with each set of exercises you do. Lie down on your left side. Elevate your legs about 20 inches higher than your head. Place a pillow in front of you to support your chest as you lean forward. Use another pillow under your right leg which is flexed for support. Have someone clap and vibrate your lower ribs beneath your right armpit, being careful not to hit your abdomen.

6. Position yourself as for Exercise 5, but this time lie on your right side with your left leg flexed. Have someone clap and vibrate your lower ribs beneath your left armpit.

When the exercises call for clapping, have your helper cup his hands, keeping his fingers and thumb close together. The sound made by the cupped hand tapping the chest must be hollow, not slapping. Have him use both hands in a uniform rhythm, keeping wrists flexible and elbows slightly bent. Continue for 1½ to 2 minutes. During clapping, always cover the chest with a gown or towel.

When exercises call for vibration, have your helper place his hands flat, directly on the percussed area. Take a deep breath. As you exhale, have your helper vibrate his arms. Repeat vibration at least 3 times. Make sure the pressure applied is forceful, but not excessive.

These exercises will help you clear your lungs of mucus. You'll need a helper. Don't forget to take deep breaths, fully expand your chest, and cough with each new position.

1. With pillows behind you, sit on a chair and lean back from your waist at a 30° angle. Have your partner clap your upper front chest just below the collarbone, one side at a time. He should stand behind you, placing one arm around your neck so that both hands fit easily on one side of your front chest.

2. Sit on the edge of your bed. Place a folded pillow on your lap or over the back of the chair and lean forward at a 30° angle, resting your arms on the pillow. Have someone clap or vibrate your upper back on the shoulder blades.

3. Lie down. Place pillows under your hips and legs to keep your legs about 16 inches

collapse. Be extra careful about using high ventilatory pressures; misused pressures can cause barotrauma of the lungs. Do everything you can to ease the psychological pressures which often cause ventilator patients to become disoriented, agitated, or even develop stress ulcers. Talk to the patient. Devise ways for him to communicate—with a child's alphabet board, or whatever. Tell him that *ventilator patients are never left unmonitored*. Check on him at least once an hour.

Stay alert for respiratory infection, falling blood pressure, stress ulcers, and airway problems. Turn the patient frequently and provide active or passive range-of-motion exercises, if permitted. As soon as he is able, get the patient out of bed and into a chair for some time each day. *An important precaution*: Make sure an Ambu bag with oxygen hookup is kept at the bedside of all patients on mechanical ventilation. If the ventilator seems to be malfunctioning, disconnect the patient and ventilate him with an Ambu bag until help arrives.

Expect to find improved arterial blood gases 15 to 30 minutes after mechanical respiration begins. Also look for corresponding improvements in resting tidal volume, vital capacity, and inspiratory force. Check for clinical signs of improved respiration: improved ventilatory distribution, blood pressure, skin perfusion, and alertness. If the patient shows no improvement, the doctor may add on PEEP (positive end expiratory pressure), a special ventilation mode, for additional respiratory support. PEEP's positive pressure prevents the collapse of small airways during exhalation and improves the distribution of gases throughout the lungs.

When to wean?
When the patient's respiratory deficit has been reversed and he can meet his metabolic demands for carbon dioxide elimination and oxygen transfer, *slowly* wean him from the respirator. Usually, a wide-bore T-piece is attached to a source of humidified O_2, such as a nebulizer. Encourage the patient to breathe through the T-piece without machine assistance for gradually lengthening periods each day, until he's free of the machine. An alternative weaning method uses IMV with the ventilator set to deliver progressively fewer machine-delivered breaths per minute until the patient is breathing on his own. Reduce his anxiety about separation from the ventilator by reassuring the patient that he can return to it if severe respiratory distress recurs.

COMA
Meeting the most challenging test

BY NANCY R. ADAMS, RN, MSN, MAJ, ANC

DO YOU CONSIDER CARING for the comatose patient frustrating, fruitless, and unrewarding. Frustrating and extremely difficult it certainly is. But fruitless and unrewarding? Not at all. Your nursing care sustains the comatose patient's life from one moment to the next. And the *quality* of this care can profoundly influence his potential for complete recovery. Yet the care is complex, because it must compensate for total dependency. Obviously, such care emphasizes respiratory status, musculoskeletal function, and skin integrity. But it includes much more: feeding, eye and mouth care, and excretory function to name but a few.

When the patient is admitted or transferred from another unit, your first priority, of course, is attention to the ABCs of resuscitation — airway, breathing, and circulation. If his cardiopulmonary status is stable, your next priority is to identify the cause of the coma — trauma, drug reactions, diabetes, CVA, or whatever. Treat a patient who has suffered head and cervical trauma as if he has spinal injuries until excluded by X-rays and neurologic examination. If he's on a backboard, keep him on it and carefully immobilize his neck. Don't turn his neck if resuscitation is necessary. Log-roll him

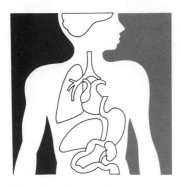

Common causes of coma
Knowing the usual causes of coma will sharpen your assessment skills and help you anticipate the necessary medical intervention.

CHEMICAL
Alcohol
Carbon dioxide and carbon
    monoxide narcosis
Anoxia
TRAUMATIC
Skull fracture
Subdural hematoma
Subarachnoid hemorrhage
Brain stem injury
INFECTIOUS
Syphilis of the CNS
Meningitis — viral or bacterial
Encephalitis
VASCULAR
Cerebral aneurysm (berry) and/or
    rupture
Cerebral tumor
Cerebral vascular lesions
Cardiac decompensation
Shock — hemorrhagic, septic,
    hypovolemic
OTHER
Diabetes
Hepatic failure
Electrolyte disorders
Deficiencies of thiamine and
    vitamin B12
Poisoning
Seizures
Uremia

during assessment so his head doesn't turn with his shoulders.

If he doesn't require assisted ventilation, he'll usually need 2 to 4 liters of oxygen per minute via nasal prongs or mask. Also evaluate the patient's level of consciousness. This is vital in order to provide a baseline for changes and cerebral status.

After initial assessment, begin baseline diagnostic studies. Usually, you'll draw blood for glucose, arterial blood gases, BUN, and electrolyte determination and tests for toxic substances (such as barbiturates). These studies can help identify hypoglycemia, drug overdose, electrolyte abnormalities, renal failure, or hypoxemia.

Next, most doctors will have you establish an I.V. line and give a bolus injection of 25 to 50 g of a 50% glucose solution. The rationale? Profound hypoglycemia can cause irreparable brain damage. Generally, you'll give alcoholic patients 100 mg of thiamine with the glucose, since they are usually deficient in thiamine, a vitamin necessary for glucose metabolism. Patients suspected of overdosing with narcotics may have already received an antidote in the emergency room. If not, try to get a urine sample by catheter before giving a narcotic antagonist. (Of course, if the patient is having severe respiratory depression, correcting that would become your first priority.) But, whenever possible, try to get the urine sample first because the urine metabolites of narcotic antagonists can't be distinguished from those produced by a narcotic.

Sometime during early treatment, you must take as complete a history as possible by interviewing the patient's relatives, acquaintances, or anyone else who accompanied him to the hospital. Ask especially about any history of alcoholism, drug use, diabetes, or seizures. If the patient has suffered trauma, ask for details of the injuries.

Check vital signs at least every 15 minutes during early treatment. If a comatose patient goes into shock, examine him closely for internal bleeding. Remember, in an adult a closed-head injury rarely causes shock. Adequate volume replacement is the most important treatment for hypovolemic shock. Albumin and other colloids will increase blood volume as efficiently as whole blood, but avoid hypotonic I.V. solutions because they tend to increase cerebral edema, often

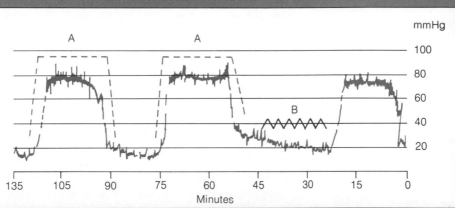

MONITORING INTRACRANIAL PRESSURE

The cranial contents—blood, brain, and cerebrospinal fluid (CSF)—fill the skull to capacity. Increased volume of any of these can be tolerated to a point. But when all available space in the skull is filled, intracranial pressure (ICP) rises sharply with any further increase in volume.

CSF production is normally 500 ml/day. But much of this CSF is reabsorbed so that the volume in the cerebrospinal cavity is maintained at only 150 ml. And normally, the brain can "autoregulate" or maintain constant blood-flow pressure levels despite systemic arterial pressure changes. However, when ICP exceeds systemic arterial pressure, inadequate cerebral perfusion causes cerebral hypoxia and may lead to brain damage or death.

How measured?
ICP and VFV (ventricular fluid volume) are measured by ventriculostomy. A catheter, via stylet, with a large-bore needle is inserted into the *right lateral* ventricle of the cerebrum, and then connected to a pressure transducer which records

pressure and volume. The result is the two waves shown above, "A" and "B" waves. The "A" wave is a plateau wave, and occurs when ICP falls within a range of 50 to 115 mmHg for 5 to 20 minutes. The "B" or baseline wave occurs when ICP falls within 20 to 40 mmHg for 5 to 20 minutes, and changes according to the patient's respirations. A "C" wave may also be identified. It corresponds to changes in arterial blood pressure. Like the B wave, it is not clinically significant.

Hypercapnia, hypoxia (PO₂ less than 50 mmHg), body position, isometric vascular contractions, increased cortical activity during REM sleep, and the Valsalva maneuver may all cause ICP to rise sharply in patients with a full cranial cavity. Because this rise can occur rapidly, watch for and report clinical signs (such as headache, forced breathing, purposeless movements, and cloudy sensorium) that coincide with the onset and peak of plateau waves. If you notice such changes, check vital signs more often. Don't wait for motor or pupillary activity, wide pulse

pressure, or bradycardia as clues to increased ICP. These are late clues that develop after a sustained plateau wave, when permanent brain damage may already have occurred. For external CSF drainage, you can connect the tubing to a collection bag. Then, frequently check the tubing for patency and make sure the fluid is flowing freely. Even during position changes, keep the patient's head at a 30° angle, and keep the drainage bag level with his head.
To prevent increases in ICP:
• Avoid flexing the patient's neck and hip when monitoring.
• When patients want to reposition themselves in bed, instruct them to move slowly and to exhale as they do so, to avoid a Valsalva maneuver.
• Discourage patient from straining at stool (a stool softener may be indicated).
• Maintain patent airway.
• Hyperventilate the patient before suctioning.
• Don't leave the catheter down longer than 10 seconds.
• Give mannitol (Osmitrol) and corticosteroids (Hydrocortisone, Cortisone) as prescribed.

Recognize the rates

Changes in respiratory rate may signal important physiologic changes. If you learn the different breath sounds and the conditions that produce them, you'll be better prepared to intervene appropriately.

EUPNEA
Normal respiration.

TACHYPNEA
Increased respiratory rate, seen in fever, for example, as the body tries to rid itself of excess heat. Respirations increase about 4 breaths a minute for every 1° F. rise in temperature above normal. They also increase with pneumonia, compensatory respiratory alkalosis, respiratory insufficiency, and lesions in the pons of the brain stem.

HYPERVENTILATION
Increased respiratory rate and depth. This follows extreme exertion, fear and anxiety, fever, hepatic coma, midbrain lesions of the brain stem, acid-base imbalances, hypercarbia, and decreased oxygen. The breathing pattern in hyperventilation: inspiration, a pause, a longer expiration, and another pause.

(continued)

present in comatose patients.

Whenever you care for a patient with a head injury never, under any circumstances, place his head lower than the rest of his body. This would push the abdominal contents against his diaphragm and interfere with breathing. It would also increase pressure on his brain and could also stimulate vasopressor receptors in his aorta and carotid arteries, causing vasoconstriction of cerebral blood vessels and cerebral ischemia. Keep the patient's head elevated 15° to 30°.

Watch intracranial pressure

The classic triad of slow pulse, increased blood pressure, and a wide pulse pressure indicates a late sign of increased intracranial pressure. Prior to these you should observe for pupillary changes, i.e., dilated pupil that reacts sluggishly or not at all to light. How to treat rising intracranial pressure? Usually with a hyperosmotic agent. It's usually given as mannitol 20%, 1 to 5 g/Kg of body weight, over 30 to 60 minutes. Mannitol moves water out of the body cells to the bloodstream where the kidneys can remove it. Such a solution sometimes contains crystals, so be careful with this infusion: Warm the container in water to dissolve the crystals. And use an infusion set with a filter, in case the solution recrystallizes.

Monitor patients carefully during hyperosmotic therapy. Watch especially for circulatory overload in elderly cardiac patients whose kidney function may be incapable of handling the increased volume.

You may also be called on to treat elevated intracranial pressure by mechanically hyperventilating the patient. That can relieve intracranial pressure because the resulting respiratory alkalosis will decrease cerebral circulation by causing cerebral vasoconstriction.

To achieve such hyperventilation, we use a Bennett MA-1 ventilator and we monitor blood gases hourly until the patient's PCO_2 reaches the desired level; afterwards, once each shift. We aim for an arterial PCO_2 of 30 mmHg. This mild alkalosis usually sees the patient through the 48- to 72-hour period typical for an episode of high intracranial pressure. Such alkalosis needs no treatment unless the PCO_2 drops significantly below 20 mmHg. Weaning from the ventilator must be gradual to allow time for restoration of normal PCO_2

levels in blood and cerebrospinal fluid. Normal P_{CO_2} levels are the patient's stimuli to breathe.

If hyperosmotic treatment or hyperventilation fails to control increasing intracranial pressure, the patient usually needs surgery to relieve it.

Monitor temperature closely

Cerebral edema is often accompanied by fever which, in turn, can increase intracranial pressure through vasodilation. To prevent this, keep the patient with cerebral edema slightly hypothermic with a cooling blanket or pad. Hypothermia decreases cerebral pressure by inducing vasoconstriction and protects the brain by lowering cerebral glucose and oxygen requirements.

At our hospital, we aim to keep such a patient's temperature at about 93° to 94° F. (33.9° to 34.4° C.). We stop cooling at about 95° F. (35° C.) because the temperature will then continue to fall another degree or two. During cooling, we check temperature rectally every 30 minutes. Taking oral temperatures is contraindicated for comatose patients. Besides, rectal probes are the easiest way to monitor temperature constantly. The probe must be accurate and working properly; then inserted into the rectum about 3 inches, angled anteriorly.

Nursing tip: Don't cool the patient down so much that he shivers. Shivering can cause an increase in intracranial pressure.

Long-term care

Your long-range goals for nursing a comatose patient are clear-cut and demanding:

• to maintain the patient in optimal physical condition

• to prevent complications arising from immobility and impaired neurologic status

• to assist the doctor in treating the underlying condition responsible for the coma.

How to achieve these goals? First by meticulous respiratory care. Respiratory failure is the most prevalent cause of death in comatose patients. Its usual cause: blockage of the airway (by a mucous plug or regurgitated stomach contents). You can minimize such aspiration and blockage by elevating the head of the patient's bed at least 30°. Place the entire bed

Recognize the rates (continued)
This pattern may be altered by certain defects and diseases. In adults, more than 20 breaths per minute is considered moderate hyperventilation; more than 30, severe.

CHEYNE-STOKES
An abnormal pattern of respiration in which cycles of hyperventilation alternate with periods of apnea. During cycles of hyperventilation (a period of 30 to 45 seconds), respirations gradually increase in rate and depth, then decrease to apnea (which lasts about 20 seconds). Cheyne-Stokes respirations may follow increased intracranial pressure, severe congestive heart failure, renal failure, meningitis, and drug overdose.

KUSSMAUL
Increased rate (more than 20 per minute) and increased depth; a panting, labored respiration seen in metabolic acidosis or renal failure.

APNEUSTIC
Prolonged, gasping inspiration, followed by extremely short, inefficient expiration, seen in lesions of the pons in the midbrain.

at an angle by putting shock blocks under the *head of the bed*. This works better than cranking up the mattress, which keeps the patient in a constant sitting position (placing excessive pressure on his buttocks). During feeding and for 30 minutes afterward, keep the head of the bed cranked up an additional 30°. This, too, will help prevent aspiration of food. If the doctor wants the patient to lie flat, keep him in a semiprone, side-lying position. Avoid letting him lie flat on his back.

Remember that the danger of aspiration is greatest during routine tube feedings. This is so because the patient regurgitates food when his stomach becomes distended. You can minimize distention by removing residual stomach contents before each feeding and subtracting this volume from the new feeding. Then, reinstill the residual contents (which contain necessary gastric juices) with the new food.

Let's look at an example. A standard feeding order calls for 250 ml of formula with 50 ml of water. If the patient's residual content was 100 ml, you would subtract 100 ml from the standard 250 ml, and feed only 150 ml of new formula with 50 ml of water. If you follow this procedure, the patient's stomach can contain no more than 300 ml at any one time and stomach contents can't build up.

Monitoring residual stomach content also helps you evaluate GI status. A consistently large or increasing residual could indicate an ileus. In such cases, watch for diminishing or absent bowel sounds. If you do find signs of ileus, notify the doctor.

An intubated comatose patient should, of course, have a cuffed endotracheal tube to protect his airway. However, unless the patient is on a ventilator, the cuff should not be inflated except during feeding and for 30 minutes afterwards.

Despite the most careful positioning and feeding, some comatose patients, particularly those with impaired cough reflexes, have recurring breathing difficulties. They tend to retain secretions, which cause obstructions and provide an ideal medium for infection. Such patients should have frequent deep tracheal suctioning to remove tenacious secretions. They should also receive IPPB treatment, percussion, and postural drainage at least once every shift.

When a comatose patient needs mechanical ventilation for longer than a week or has difficulty with clearing airway secretions, the doctor will usually perform a tracheostomy.

The patient will afterwards require humidified oxygen to maintain arterial PO_2 at about 90 mm Hg. If he doesn't need oxygen to maintain good arterial oxygen levels, use a nebulizer to keep secretions thin and to avoid crusting, irritation, and erosion of his airway mucosa.

Remove secretions by careful suctioning, using sterile technique. Just before suctioning, hyperventilate (hyperoxygenate) the patient and instill 5 ml of sterile saline. *Nursing tip:* Limit suctioning time to not more than 10 to 15 seconds — the amount of time you can comfortably hold your own breath. If you can't remove all secretions in this time, ventilate the patient again and repeat the suctioning. Change the dressings around the tracheostomy at least once each shift; more often, if they become soiled or wet. Be sure to clean the stoma and check it for changes in appearance.

Watch every intubated, comatose patient carefully to ensure that his tracheostomy tube remains clear. Arrange his bedclothes so he can't accidentally move them and block the tube. Watch for tachycardia, increased blood pressure, absence of chest movement, and absent breath sounds—all signs of airway obstruction.

Give nasal passages scrupulous care to prevent dried secretions from forming an obstruction. About twice a day, swab the nares with a cotton-tipped applicator moistened with saline. You'll find a nebulizer useful for keeping secretions thin and avoiding crusting irritation and erosion of mucosa in patients not intubated. (Always obtain the doctor's permission before inserting applicators in the nose or ears of any patient who has had a craniotomy or brain injury.)

Notify the doctor immediately if you notice any bleeding or fluid drainage from the patient's nose or ears. To determine if the fluid contains cerebrospinal fluid (CSF), test it for glucose. A positive test indicates CSF. Bloody drainage that contains CSF will not clot and leaves a distinctive mark on bedclothes: The outer ring of the stain is lighter because CSF is less dense and spreads farther than blood.

Protect skin and muscles
Because most comatose patients can't move, their nursing care must include measures to prevent skin breakdown from prolonged surface pressure, musculoskeletal atrophy, and fixation of extremities in nonfunctional positions. Such mea-

ONE GOOD TURN

Since turning the comatose or bedridden patient plays such an important part in preventing complications, try using this charting schedule. Place it in full view over the patient's bed for the best continuity of care. For handy reference, you'll want to color-code the time schedule for each shift.

7 A.M. TO 3 P.M. SHIFT		3 P.M. TO 11 P.M. SHIFT		11 P.M. TO 7 A.M. SHIFT	
8 a.m.	Supine or semi-Fowler's	4 p.m.	Supine or semi-Fowler's	12 mn.	Supine or semi-Fowler's
10 a.m.	Right lateral	6 p.m.	Right lateral	2 a.m.	Right lateral
12 n.	Left lateral	8 p.m.	Left lateral	4 a.m.	Left lateral
2 p.m.	Prone (if not contraindicated)	10 p.m.	Prone (if not contraindicated)	6 a.m.	Prone (if not contraindicated)

sures include:

• An air mattress: Put one on the bed as soon as the comatose patient is admitted. Never place turning sheets or disposable linen-savers between the patient and the mattress — the extra covering increases pressure on the skin, negating the advantages of the air mattress. Pillows and blanket rolls are usually sufficient for proper positioning.

• A strict turning schedule that specifies positions: Make a card that specifies turning times and positions and place it over the patient's bed. Such a card might specify: 2 p.m., right side; 4 p.m., left side; 6 p.m., supine; and so forth.

• Meticulous skin care: If the patient needs a cooling pad, maintaining skin integrity is more difficult. Turn such a patient at least every 2 hours. Treat any areas of redness and breakdown aggressively as soon as they appear.

• Range-of-motion exercises for arms, legs, and feet every nursing shift: Use lightweight plastic splints to maintain functional positioning of arms and legs, and to prevent wristdrop and footdrop if the patient is not spastic. Remove the splints every 4 hours to inspect underlying skin. Even softly padded splints can cause skin breakdown in a patient with decerebrate or decorticate postures. Properly fitting high-top basketball sneakers and thick cotton socks work well in preventing foot-drop. Make sure they're not laced tightly and fit properly, or decreased circulation and/or pressure sores can develop. Alternate them off and on every 2 to 4 hours, along with your turning schedule.

Special eye care

Because their corneal reflex is usually diminished or absent, comatose patients need special eye care to prevent corneal abrasions and possible blindness. Every 4 hours, remove dried secretions from their eyes with sterile gauze moistened with normal saline, and instill methylcellulose eyedrops (artificial tears). If their eyes tend to stay open and corneal reflex is completely absent, consult an ophthalmologist about inserting eye-shields. Or keep their eyelids closed with Steri-strips, eyepads, or shields, changing them every 4 hours when you clean their eyes.

Mouth care

I usually begin mouth care by brushing the patient's teeth and cleaning his gums with a padded tongue blade soaked in mouthwash. I always get someone to help me rinse the patient's mouth; one person irrigates while the other suctions. I find it best to use a 20-cc syringe filled with 15 ml of mouthwash and 5 ml of hydrogen peroxide. I put a 2-inch plastic I.V. catheter on the end of the syringe to provide a soft, flexible irrigating tip.

You might prefer to use a Water Pik for cleaning the patient's mouth. Position the patient on his side so that any liquid not immediately suctioned will drain out. After cleaning, and throughout the day every 2 hours, lubricate the patient's lips with lemon-glycerin swabs to prevent drying and cracking. Avoid using lemon and glycerin or any combination containing oil *inside* the mouth, because aspirated particles may cause respiratory problems.

Oral intubation may hamper proper mouth care. Try to insert a bite block or an oral airway to prevent the patient from biting down on the intubation tube. Change his mouthpiece each shift when you clean his mouth.

Sometimes you'll be unable to open the patient's mouth at all, because his jaw is rigid. Then, you're forced to limit mouth care to cleaning gums and brushing teeth. Later, if you can open the mouth after a patient has been without oral hygiene for a prolonged time, take care not to dislodge any collected particles that might be aspirated. The uvula, particularly, tends to collect dried secretions.

Some comatose patients clench their jaws and grind their teeth. To protect their teeth and tongue, consult an oral surgeon to provide a bite block appliance. The tape holding the endotracheal tube often gets wet during mouth care and must be changed. This procedure also takes two people: One holds the tube in place while the other does the taping. To make the tape stick, apply tincture of benzoin to the skin. Shave male patients daily before taping. Listen for breath sounds on both sides after retaping to make sure that the tube is positioned properly above the carina.

Feeding methods vary
The comatose patient needs a minimum of 1800 calories of commercially prepared canned food in divided feedings every 3 or 4 hours. Or, sometimes the doctor may prefer continuous feedings administered by gravity drip or motorized roller pump.

Feed by nasogastric or gastrostomy tubes, or by I.V. hyperalimentation? Many institutions prefer the nasogastric tube — it's usually already in place to empty the stomach, and the other methods have important disadvantages. For example, gastrostomy feeding requires surgery to establish and close the openings. I.V. feeding can cause phlebitis, infection, metabolic problems, and also interfere with turning the patient. But nasogastric feeding isn't problem-free either. Tube feedings are highly concentrated and tend to extract water from the intracellular fluid into the GI tract. This can lead to dehydration (decreased urine output, elevated temperature, soft and sunken eyeballs, cool pale skin, poor skin turgor, low blood pressure, and an increased pulse rate). To avoid such dehydration, increase the amount of water instilled after the feeding. (Following food and medications with water also helps keep the nasogastric tube clear.)

Because comatose patients are vulnerable to stress ulcers, they often receive prophylactic antacids instilled via the nasogastric tube. So do patients receiving steroids. After giving an antacid, remember to flush the tube with some water, to prevent antacid residue from obstructing the tube.

Monitor excretions
All comatose patients should have a daily rectal exam. Check for fecal impaction or inadequate emptying, and remove retained stools manually. Start patients with hard stools on a stool softener or glycerin suppositories. Hard stools may indicate inadequate fluid intake; diarrhea may indicate poor absorption of tube feeding, fecal impaction, or too rapidly administered tube feedings. Have all stools checked for occult blood, a possible sign of stress ulcers.

The size of the eyes
Because the oculomotor nerve arises from the brain stem, the pupillary activity it controls provides an excellent gauge of brain stem function. Normal pupils are the same size and react symmetrically to light. Use the chart above to measure pupil size accurately.

Unequal pupil sizes suggest local compression, brain stem damage, or increased intracranial pressure. If one pupil is considerably larger than the other, report this to the doctor at once. Without immediate intervention, such a patient may die.

To test pupillary reflex to light and consensual reaction (the response of one pupil when light is flashed in the other), reduce the light in the room. Then, as you cover one of the patient's eyes, shine a bright beam of light into the other. Note any sluggish or unequal reaction as well as any unusual eye movements.

Watch urinary output carefully. Many patients with intra-cranial pathology develop diabetes insipidus because of interference with the release of vasopressin from the posterior pituitary. This deficiency can raise urinary output to more than 10 liters a day. Notify the doctor if the patient's output exceeds 200 ml per hour for 2 consecutive hours, as volume depletion, hypernatremia, or prerenal azotemia can occur.

Dried secretions may cause infections if allowed to accumulate around the urethral meatus. Prevent this by cleaning this site once each shift, or more often if secretions accumulate. Clean the meatus with sterile gauze that has been soaked in a soap solution, then apply an antiseptic ointment.

Once the patient begins to resume control of basic functions — such as eating, coughing on command, and assisting in turning — consider removing the catheter. But first, have a urologist examine the patient to determine his bladder capacity and ability to initiate voiding. When the patient is ready, you can remove the catheter (without any preliminary routine of clamping and unclamping of the catheter). Most doctors no longer consider this routine worthwhile. If the patient develops a spastic bladder and voids small amounts frequently, he may need an antispasmodic.

Assessing neurologic status

Evaluate the patient's neurologic status daily so you can accurately take changes into account.

When reporting your neurologic assessment, avoid nonspecific phrases (such as "no improvement noted" or "remains unresponsive") and ambiguous labels (such as "stuporous" or "obtunded"). Instead, use descriptive phrases that specify the level of consciousness, pattern of breathing, size and reactivity of pupils, and skeletal muscle responses (see margin, this page).

Coordinate your definitions for neurologic status with other members of the staff so everyone uses the same word to mean the same thing. Record your assessment daily. Such documentation will provide serial observations for comparison and make significant changes readily apparent. A good flow sheet will present this information in a handy, easily understood format.

Watch for any unusual movements, and clearly describe

Stages of consciousness

Use these terms to evaluate and describe your patient's level of consciousness.

ALERT — The patient is awake and fully conscious, oriented to time, place, and person, and responsive to commands and stimuli.

DROWSY
—*Lethargic:* The patient responds slowly and selectively to stimuli, ignoring some altogether. He falls asleep easily.
—*Obtunded:* The patient responds appropriately when stimulated but otherwise sleeps deeply.

STUPOROUS — The patient responds with purposeful movement only to vigorous and in some cases painful stimuli. Otherwise his thinking is slow, confused, and disoriented. He may hallucinate.

COMATOSE — The patient does not respond voluntarily to external stimuli such as pain. He may retain reflex muscle contraction. In cases of deep coma, depending on the etiology, even these responses may be absent. Painful stimuli may produce changes in respiratory patterns or decerebrate or decorticate movement.

A rigid response

When you test motor responses during a neurologic assessment, remember to notice the position your patient assumes. If he lies in one of the four positions shown here, he will have cerebral dysfunction. The first figure—where all extremities are rigidly extended and the arms are hyperpronated—indicates a lesion of the cerebrum between the midbrain and the pons. This position is called decerebrate rigidity.

The other three figures show decorticate rigidity, indicating a lesion above the brain stem to the pyramidal motor tract. In a supine posture, the legs extend and the arms flex as shown in Figure 2. If you turn the patient's head to the right, his right arm may relax but his left arm will flex. The opposite will happen if you turn his head to the left. In either case the legs will remain hyperextended.

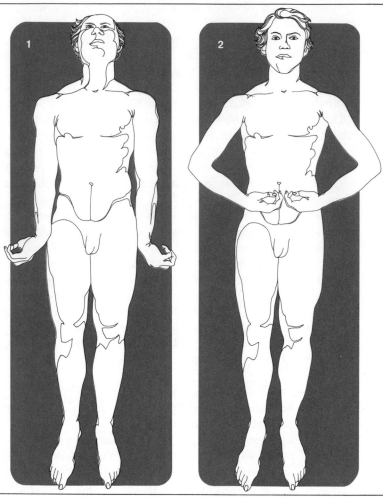

them. For example, decorticate or decerebrate rigidity may occur spontaneously or in response to pain. In decorticate movement, which accompanies damage above the brain stem to the corticospinal (pyramidal) motor tract, the patient's legs are stiffly extended and his arms sharply flexed on his chest. In decerebrate posturing that occurs with upper brain stem damage, all his extremities are rigidly extended and his arms hyperpronated. Sometimes fragments or combinations of these responses occur.

Watch for unusual movements similar to the behavior of a young infant, such as reflex sucking or grasping. Avoid mistaking these for voluntary responses: Always report them. Yawning, vomiting, or hiccoughing can occur with damage to certain lower brain stem areas. Some patients may have flaccid extremities without movement. Carefully report any abnormalities you find.

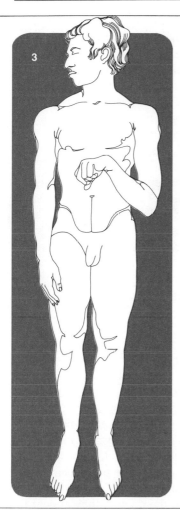

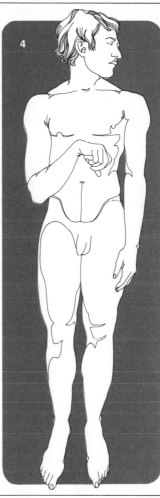

The patient may assume any of these postures spontaneously or in response to a painful stimulus.

After you've evaluated the patient's position, it's a good idea to test for a Babinski sign. This foot reflex is normal in infants under 18 months, but after that time it indicates pyramidal tract dysfunction. To do this test, first tell the patient that you're going to stroke the sole of his foot, and ask him not to move while you do so. Then, rub upward along the outer edge of each sole with a fairly sharp object, such as a key or the top of a pen.

Normally, the response should be a downward bending of the patient's big toe. If the big toe bends upward instead, this is a positive Babinski sign. While making this test, don't stroke all the way across the ball of the foot. This may be uncomfortable and make the patient pull his foot away.

Also evaluate seizure activity, another important part of neurologic assessment. An estimated 2% to 5% of patients with closed-head injuries develop focal or generalized seizures. After such seizure, report the parts of the body involved, type and duration of movement, order of spread, changes in respirations, and incontinency of bladder or bowel.

When the doctor prescribes phenytoin sodium (Dilantin) for seizures, remember that oral administration is best. (Dilantin is available as a suspension.) I.V. administration may be dangerous because this drug has a cardiac depressant action and can cause lethal arrhythmias and hypotension. Moreover it ususally precipitates in solutions when added to an I.V. However, some institutions do give Dilantin intravenously by slow push over 5 minutes, followed by flush with normal saline solution. Avoid intramuscular administration. It has the disadvantage of sometimes producing granulomas of crystals within the muscle.

Consider psychosocial needs

The comatose patient's physical needs are so overwhelming that his psychosocial needs and those of his family may be neglected. These needs aren't greatly different from those of any seriously ill patient, except in one respect — a tendency toward poorer communication between patient, family, and those providing care. In my experience, the greatest communication barrier between staff and family grows out of the uncertain prognosis. In most cases, no one can predict whether or not the patient will come out of the coma. That uncertainty can build so much tension that cooperation becomes difficult. However, I've noticed that when the staff explains the details of the care and allows the family to help as much as possible, this barrier between family and staff comes tumbling down. Then, even if the patient doesn't recover, the high quality of care he received is a great comfort to his family.

The communication barrier between staff and patient results when the staff assumes the patient is oblivious to his surroundings. But remember: Just because the patient doesn't respond, don't assume that he doesn't think, feel, or hear. He may be acutely aware of what's going on even though he can't show that he is. So, say nothing in his presence that you don't want him to hear, and keep his environment peaceful and quiet. Tell him what is happening when you give physical care, even though he gives no indication that he hears or understands. Repeatedly, we have seen patients who, after recovery, could recall details of the care they received while in profound coma. Some patients in coma first begin to make contact with their environment in response to conversation directed to them when they appear to be totally unresponsive.

Think of each of these patients as a "what if" patient. What if he wakes up tomorrow and remembers everything you did for him? Many of these patients do, and when they do, you'll be more than repaid for all your caring.

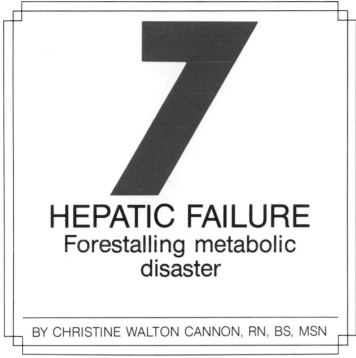

7

HEPATIC FAILURE
Forestalling metabolic disaster

BY CHRISTINE WALTON CANNON, RN, BS, MSN

THE PHRASE "CRITICALLY ILL" is never more appropriate than when applied to the patient with liver failure—a condition that adversely affects every vital function. Fortunately, it's not one you're called upon to manage every day. But when you do, the quality of your nursing skills can profoundly influence whether or not, or how soon, the patient succumbs to this metabolic disaster. How can skilled nursing intervention help patients with liver failure? Mainly by promptly recognizing developing encephalopathy and by combatting its progression...by knowing how to control the gastrointestinal bleeding so common in these patients...and by knowing ways to inhibit the breakdown of protein and other sources of excessive ammonia accumulation—the immediate cause of hepatic enccphalopathy.

Of course, knowing what to do about liver failure requires first that you know what it is; what kinds of patients are likely to develop it; and what are its early symptoms and signs.

A late development
By the time liver failure has become obvious in its characteristic symptoms and signs, it's already in a late, dangerously

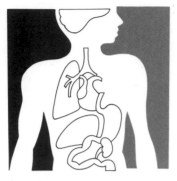

Causes of liver failure
- hepatitis (viral, fulminant, or chronic)
- gastrointestinal bleeding (also a complication)
- uremia
- infections
- toxic reactions to drugs (antidepressants, halothane and related anesthetics, tetracyclines, cinchophen, zoxazolamine, paracetamol, diuretics, analgesics, hypnotics and sedatives; carbon tetrachloride and other chemicals, poisonous mushrooms, and alcohol)
- biliary disease
- chronically inadequate liver cell oxygenation or nutrition (as in chronic congestive heart failure and malnutrition), and rarely...
- fulminant Wilson's disease
- toxemia of pregnancy
- Reye's syndrome
- genetic disorders of urea cycle enzymes

advanced stage. This is so because the liver has a large reserve capacity and needs only 10% to 20% of functioning tissue to sustain life.

Hepatic failure does sometimes occur rapidly and dramatically, as in fulminant hepatitis, in which massive liver necrosis rapidly leads to coma and death because liver regeneration can't proceed fast enough to support hepatic function. Most often, however, it develops slowly, for example as a result of long chronic hepatitis and cirrhosis often as a result of alcohol abuse.

Alcohol is the implicated toxic agent in at least 30% of all cases of hepatic failure: It also increases the liver's vulnerability to other toxic agents.

How cirrhosis happens

When liver tissue becomes necrotic, much of it is eventually replaced by connective scar tissue. Bands of such scar tissue subdivide the liver into small, irregular nodules. This diffuse, chronic overgrowth of scar tissue, along with liver-cell destruction and nodule regeneration has generally been called cirrhosis. This cirrhotic process inhibits blood flow into the liver. And it compresses and detours capillary blood flow within the liver. When it markedly impedes flow of blood into the liver (via the portal venous system), portal venous pressures rise with sluggish flow in major venous trunks and portal hypertension results. Eventually, blood, unable to enter the liver, distends and may rupture the thin-walled vessels of the stomach, esophagus, and lower rectum (where portal and general venous circulation join).

In Jim Greenwood, cirrhosis was accelerated by refusal to cooperate with treatment. Mr. Greenwood, 37 years old, was brought to the emergency department with profuse rectal bleeding. He complained of feeling very weak, and had just not been feeling well for months. He had quit his job as an assembly line worker 5 months before and had spent the interim relaxing, tanning himself, and drinking beer. He added that he really was not eating much, although his "beer belly" never seemed to get smaller. Not surprisingly, we found his "beer belly" to be obvious ascites on clinical examination. When we asked Mr. Greenwood about any past history of liver disease, he admitted that he'd been "into drugs" 5 years before and that he'd had three separate episodes of "yellow jaundice," but had recovered each time without medical help. During each episode of jaundice, he had severe anorexia, lost 10 to 15 lbs., and had some upper right quadrant abdominal pain.

The admitting doctor's diagnosis: portal cirrhosis (diffuse hepatic fibrosis) due to postnecrotic scarring following severe viral hepatitis. Presumably, chronic alcohol ingestion and a protein-deficient diet further damaged his liver cells, leading to portal hypertension and hemorrhage of rectal varices. At admission, his severe ascites made palpation of the liver and spleen very difficult. (Later, after we'd reduced his ascites with careful fluid management, percussion showed that both liver and spleen were markedly enlarged; palpation showed that the liver edge was smooth, firm, and nontender.) Inspection of the skin revealed overt jaundice, spider telangiectases (small, dilated blood vessels resulting from an increase in circulating estrogen in cirrhosis), loss of body hair, and gynecomastia, and tortuous epigastric vessels (caput medusae) radiating from the umbilicus toward the xiphoid and rib margins. The latter reflects abdominal collaterals, a helpful sign of portal hypertension. Mr. Greenwood's rectal bleeding was attributed to ruptured venous channels. Panendoscopy revealed esophageal and gastric varices.

In caring for Mr. Greenwood, we watched constantly for additional rectal bleeding, for occult blood in the stools, and for hematemesis and melena. Why so much emphasis on bleeding? The patient with cirrhosis tends to bleed easily because his liver fails to make sufficient amounts of the clotting factors. The liver needs vitamin K to make prothrombin. But absorption of vitamin K depends (because it's a fat-soluble vitamin) on adequate production of bile salts by the liver. Thus, when liver function is inadequate, prothrombin time tends to increase, as Mr. Greenwood's did. Also involved in his case: ability to convert amino acids into plasma proteins leading to a low plasma albumin level. A low albumin level, of course, reduces the blood's osmotic pressure and its ability to pull fluid from the tissues. The result: ascites.

Enzyme tests

To determine the severity of hepatic failure, we gave Mr. Greenwood a series of enzyme tests. Because the hepatic cells release certain enzymes into the circulation, measuring

THE NORMAL LIVER: AN INSIDE LOOK

- The liver is normally located in the upper abdomen under the diaphragm, with its greatest mass to the right of midline.
- It has 4 lobes: the falciform ligament separates the small left lobe from the much larger right lobe—which is, itself, divided into the right lobe proper, the quadrate lobe, and the caudate lobe.
- The liver's surface is normally smooth, superiorly convex, and inferiorly concave.
- Total blood flow is usually about 1500 ml per minute.
- Blood enters the liver via two major vessels: the portal vein drains the digestive tract and spleen; the hepatic artery supplies richly oxygenated blood from the aorta. These two vessels, along with lymphatic vasculature and bile ducts, branch repeatedly, delivering blood to sinusoids next to the liver's functional units—the lobules.
- Phagocytic cells, lining the sinusoids, engulf foreign particles and bacteria as the blood flows through the sinusoids to the central vein of each lobule.
- Then the blood recollects within the liver, continuing to the hepatic veins.
- Within the liver, bile capillaries drain into the bile ducts which then join to form the hepatic duct. The hepatic duct converges with the cystic duct from the gallbladder to form the common bile duct.
- The liver aids digestion by secreting bile, an essential for the breakdown of fats. Bile is made up of water, inorganic salts, bilirubin (the bile pigment derived from hemoglobin breakdown, bile acids (products of cholesterol breakdown), cholesterol, alkaline phosphatase, and mucin.

Liver cell plate
As shown, the liver is thought to be made up of plates, usually one cell thick. These form irregular, spongelike, cellular walls connected to each other via interlocking tunnels, called lacunae. These lacunae contain the liver capillaries, the sinusoids; their endothelial lining is formed by Kupffer's cells. Individual cells of the liver vary greatly in shape and size, depending on their position in the plate.

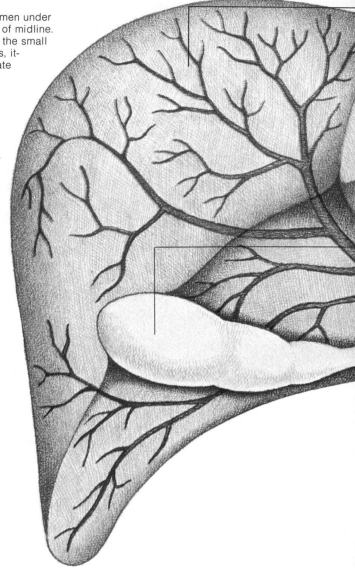

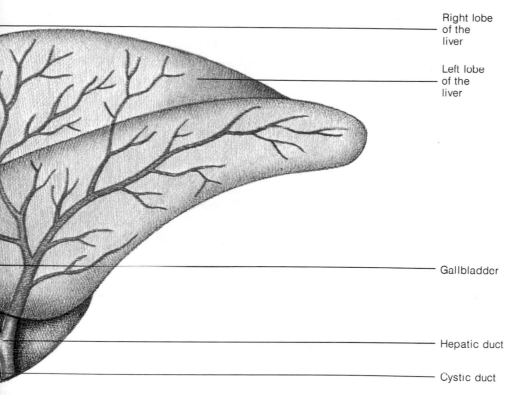

Right lobe
of the
liver

Left lobe
of the
liver

Gallbladder

Hepatic duct

Cystic duct

LIVER CELL PLATE

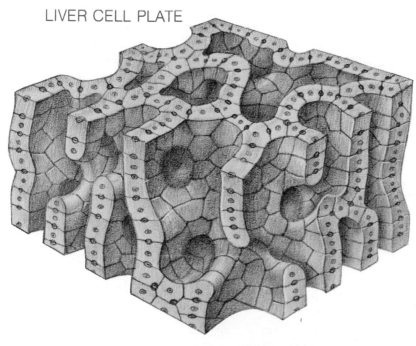

Many metabolic faces
The liver is said to perform over 500 separate metabolic functions including…
• *formation and excretion of bile salts*—essential for absorption and digestion of fats and fat-soluble vitamins in the intestine.
• *conjugation and excretion of bile pigment.* Bilirubin, the main bile pigment, is a metabolic end-product of hemolysis.
• *metabolism and storage of carbohydrates* as glycogen.
• *synthesis of serum proteins* (albumin, alpha and beta globulins, but not gamma globulins); of *blood clotting factors* (fibrinogen; prothrombin; factors V, VII, VIII, IX, and X; and vitamin K—a necessary cofactor in the synthesis of factors II, V, IX, and X); and of *urea*—formed exclusively in the liver by deamination of amino acids and bacterial action.
• *storage of amino acids and fats.*
• *synthesis and excretion of cholesterol.*
• *hydrolysis of triglycerides, cholesterol, phospholipids, and lipoproteins* to fatty acids and glycerol.
• *storage of minerals* (copper and iron) *and fat-soluble vitamins* (A, D, E, K, B12).
• *metabolism of steroids* (inactivation and excretion of aldosterone, glucocorticoids, estrogen, progesterone, and testosterone).
• *detoxification of potentially harmful drugs.*
• *filtration of blood.* Backed-up blood from venae cavae (right heart failure) rests in the liver sinusoids, where phagocytic action of Kupffer's cells removes bacteria and debris.

these enzymes gives the most direct index of liver damage. These enzymes include:
• *serum alkaline phosphatase,* a heat-stable liver enzyme found in its heat labile form in the bone, but in liver disease, it elevates and reflects impaired liver function (normal—30 to 85 international units/ml)
• *serum 5 nucleotidase*, found solely within the hepatocytes (normal—5 to 40 units/ml)
• *serum glutamic oxalacetic transaminase* (SGOT), found in the myocardium, skeletal muscles, and kidneys, as well as the liver (normal—5 to 40 units/ml);
• *serum glutamic pyruvic transaminase* (SGPT), specific to liver-cell injury (normal—5 to 35 units/ml)
• *total serum bilirubin*, the amount of pigment formed from the breakdown of hemoglobin that is normally converted by the liver and dumped into the digestive tract. Bilirubin rises markedly with hepatitis; minimally with cirrhosis (normal—0.3 to 1.0 mg)
• *lactic dehydrogenase* (LDH), an enzyme released during glycolytic activity that may be present with many diseases (normal—90 to 200 units/ml).

Mr. Greenwood's enzyme levels were moderately elevated. His SGPT was 110 units/ml and his alkaline phosphatase, 25 units/ml. (If these same enzymes had been measured during any of his episodes of hepatitis, they'd surely have been much higher.) His total serum bilirubin was 3 mg % per 100 ml. His routine lab data also included CBC, electrolytes, BUN, and creatinine. Later, his blood ammonia levels were also checked.

Naturally, monitoring Mr. Greenwood's vital signs during his episode of rectal bleeding was very important. However, once the bleeding stopped, controlling his ascites took priority. As you know, renal failure often complicates hepatic failure. So to keep track of fluid status, we weighed him daily and restricted his sodium intake to 500 mg daily, and protein to 40 g daily. After 3 days of such restriction, Mr. Greenwood had lost a mere 3 lbs, so his doctor prescribed spironolactone 100 mg daily and 2 days later added furosemide 80 mg. At last, this combination of diet, fluid restriction, and diuretics began to bring his ascites under control as he lost 4 lbs of fluid in 24 hours.

To reduce resistant ascites, the patient might receive salt-poor albumin (25 g I.V. daily) to assist diuresis. But Mr. Greenwood's ascites came under control without it. We worried about diuresing Mr. Greenwood too rapidly because electrolyte or acid-base imbalances (especially hypokalemia and alkalosis) might provoke hepatic encephalopathy.

What happens in hepatic failure is that diuretics, vomiting, diarrhea, and the diuresis due to secondary aldosteronism, collectively lead to low serum potassium. This, in turn, draws cellular potassium into the blood, in exchange for a flow of hydrogen ions back into the cells. The result is metabolic alkalosis and hypokalemia—both of which increase blood ammonia levels and favor absorption of ammonia across the blood-brain barrier. But the failing liver can't adequately convert this ammonia into urea for excretion. A patient in this condition needs supplementary potassium regulated according to the patient's electrolyte levels. If he doesn't get it, he's likely to develop hepatic coma.

Portal hypertension life-threatening

When Mr. Greenwood's panendoscopy confirmed esophageal and gastric varices, we knew his cirrhosis had reached a life-threatening stage, the result of portal hypertension. To relieve portal hypertension, the doctor considered a surgical shunt—to relieve pressure in the portal system and thereby in the distended esophageal, gastric, and hemorrhoidal veins by bypassing the liver. This would help relieve the varices and ascites but could induce encephalopathy. Such bypass would dump ammonia and toxins into the systemic circulation causing blood ammonia to rise. It could also precipitate hemorrhage by reducing clotting factors released into the bloodstream. And it could aggravate liver failure by reducing liver perfusion with oxygen and nutrients. For the moment, the question of surgery was only academic anyway. Mr. Greenwood was in no condition for it. He had to be prepared for it physically and psychologically. His doctor prescribed strict bedrest to lessen metabolic demands on the liver; a low-protein diet (40 g daily) to decrease liver metabolic workload and blood ammonia level; fluid and salt restriction to control ascites; and twice weekly injections of vitamin K to support

Stages of encephalopathy

Stage 1—PRODROMAL:
mild confusion, euphoria or
depression, vacant stare,
inappropriate laughter, forgetful-
ness, inability to concentrate,
slow mentation, slurred speech,
untidiness, lethargy, belligerence, minimal asterixis.
    Watch carefully for these
subtle signs. You won't neces-
sarily see all of them at once.

Stage 2—IMPENDING:
obvious obtundation, aberrant
behavior, definite asterixis,
constructional apraxia.
    To test for asterixis (flapping
tremors) have patient raise
both arms with forearms fixed
and fingers extended. To test for
constructional apraxia, keep a
serial record of patient's
handwriting and figure construction.

Stage 3—STUPOROUS:
marked confusion, stupor (but
patient arousable), incoherent
speech, asterixis, noisiness,
abusiveness, violence, definitely
abnormal EEG.
    Restraints may be necessary
at this stage. Do not sedate
the patient; a sedative could be
fatal.

Stage 4—COMATOSE:
coma, patient unarousable,
responds only to painful stimuli,
no asterixis, positive Babinski,
hepatic fetor (musty sweetish
odor), elevated blood ammonia
level.
    Degree of hepatic fetor corre-
lates with degree of somnolence
and confusion.

residual hepatic function.

Counseling important

To encourage Mr. Greenwood's cooperation with treatment,
we told him how serious his illness was and explained everything in his treatment plan and what we hoped it would ac-
·complish. In fact, we gave this explanation repeatedly, but he
seemed determined not to hear or understand anything we
said. Throughout his hospitalization, he continued to deny
his illness. At the time of his discharge, he had refused surgery
but promised to consider it.

Tragically, Mr. Greenwood continued to deny his illness
after discharge just as he had done before and continued to
seek refuge in drugs and alcohol—both toxic to his small
remnant of liver function. He disregarded his diet, his medications, and his need for rest. Within a week after discharge,
his ascites had recurred, and he began hemorrhaging from
both esophageal and gastric varices. Again he was rushed to
the hospital. At admission, our first priority was to control the
hemorrhage and concomitant hypovolemic shock. We began
immediate blood replacement, and placed a Sengstaken-
·Blakemore tube for aspiration of the stomach and iced saline
lavage and to apply direct pressure on the hemorrhaging areas
(see insert pages 140-141). We added Levophed to the iced
saline for additional vasoconstricting effect and held it in the
stomach by clamping the tube for 15 minutes before draining.
The cold saline with levophed bitartrate (Levophed) did help
to slow his bleeding. If it hadn't, we'd have used an intravenous
or arterial infusion of vasopressin (Pitressin). Intravenous Pitressin lowers portal blood flow and pressure. It also lowers
cardiac output dependent on dosage (so use cautiously in cardiac disease). Infusion of vasopressors directly into the superior mesenteric artery via a catheter inserted through the
femoral artery may also help control bleeding. During such
infusion, the patient must be carefully monitored for onset of
metabolic acidosis and checked for intestinal cramping,
suggestive of bowel ischemia. Either of these effects call for
lowering the vasopressor dose.

·Dreaded complication

After 4 hours, we had Mr. Greenwood's bleeding under control. Now that he was hemodynamically stable, our next prior-

---

STERILIZE THE BOWEL FOR AMMONIA DETOXIFICATION

Though it's impossible to really sterilize the bowel, you can greatly decrease its bacterial population, prevent bacteria from converting amino acids into ammonia and so control ammonia levels, with . . .

NEOMYCIN (a broad-spectrum antibiotic used to suppress bacterial flora of the GI tract).

* For the first 24 hours give 100 mg/Kg in 4 divided doses. Then lower to 50 mg/Kg daily in 4 divided doses. Record the dose. Make sure daily dose doesn't exceed 3 g.
* Make sure that urine, blood, and audiometric tests are given before and during extended neomycin therapy.
* Give neomycin on time. If you miss a scheduled dose, notify the doctor.
* Alert the rest of the staff that the patient is on bowel prep.
* Closely observe the patient for possible nephrotoxic (oliguria, anuria, flank pain, fever, increased white blood count) and ototoxic (decreased hearing) effects.
* Monitor vital signs, fluid intake and output, and electrolyte and BUN lab values.
* Be cautious with concurrent use of other ototoxic and nephrotoxic antimicrobial drugs during neomycin therapy.
* Avoid concurrent administration of diuretics—edecrin, furosemide—which may cause cumulative adverse effects.

SORBITOL (used to provoke osmotic diarrhea, to evacuate nitrogenous substrates).

* Administer as high an enema as possible.
* Use large quantities of water.

LACTULOSE (a synthetic disaccharide that decreases colonic bacterial action).

* Give a dose of 2 to 3 tablespoonfuls (30 to 45 ml) 3 to 4 times daily until stools become semisolid.
* Adjust the dosage daily to produce 2 or 3 soft stools.
* Give lactulose in fruit juice or water to weaken its distasteful sweetness.
* Do not give any other laxative during lactulose treatment.
* Store at room temperature.

---

ity was to prevent the onset of encephalopathy—a potentially fatal complication of hemorrhage in the cirrhotic patient. The root of hepatic encephalopathy is ammonia intoxication; its clinical effect, severe brain dysfunction. It follows rising blood ammonia levels resulting from excessive nitrogenous intake, fluid and electrolyte imbalances, sepsis, end-stage liver failure with azotemia, excessive accumulation of nitrogenous body wastes (from constipation or gastrointestinal hemorrhage); and, bacterial action on protein and urea to form ammonia.

To keep ahead of this complication, we carefully monitored arterial blood ammonia level. It was definitely rising, so we watched carefully for signs of nervous system involvement. We checked his neurologic status every 4 hours, and found progressive signs of encephalopathy (see opposite page) with each check. Mr. Greenwood was clearly in stage II of hepatic encephalopathy when we noticed asterixis ("flapping tremors" exhibited when arms are stretched out and held still while wrists are hyperextended and fingers are separated); apraxia (inability to construct simple figures); and inability to use an object in spite of knowing its name and function.

To stop progression of encephalopathy, our plan of treatment called for eliminating ammonigenic material from the GI tract by continued aspiration of blood from the stomach; catharsis (Sorbitol) to produce an osmotic diarrhea; neomycin sulfate (Neomycin) enemas t.i.d. to suppress the bacterial flora in the GI tract (preventing them from converting amino acids into ammonia); and lactulose (Cephulac) to suppress bacterial elaboration of ammonia. Lactulose is helpful because bacterial enzymes in the colon convert lactulose into lactic acid, making the colon too acid for bacterial growth. This rise in the number of available hydrogen ions encourages conversion of absorbable NH_3 to poorly absorbed NH_4 which can then be excreted in the stool.

After 2 days of this treatment Mr. Greenwood's encephalopathy began to improve. His flapping tremor disappeared and his sensorium was near normal. We discontinued the bowel regimen and IV infusions, but continued his special diet—low protein, high carbohydrate, and supplemental thiamine and multivitamins. His vital signs continued to improve gradually to normal levels. He remained stable and after 5 days was transferred to the medical/surgical floor for continued treatment and preparation for portacaval shunt. His longterm prospects? Mr. Greenwood was by no means out of the woods. His chances for survival would depend—as they do in such patients—on his willingness to abstain from alcohol and to eat a nutritious, well-balanced diet.

SKILLCHECK 2

1. Patients in renal failure need to reduce their protein intake. What is the minimum daily protein intake required for tissue repair and maintenance?
a) 40 g daily
b) 30 g daily
c) 20 g daily
d) 10 g daily

2. Which of the following is *not* an advantage of peritoneal dialysis?
a) It doesn't require complex machinery and specialized personnel.
b) Heparinization isn't necessary.
c) It's the most rapid and efficient method of dialysis.
d) It can be done immediately.

3. Which of the following drugs would *not* be used in treating cardiogenic shock?
a) Vasodilators
b) Diuretics
c) Vasoconstrictors
d) All of the above
e) A and B only

4. You're caring for 58-year-old Roger Callan, a cardiogenic shock patient who's had a Swan-Ganz pulmonary artery line inserted. While observing the oscilloscope, you notice a right ventricular wave pattern. What should you do?
a) Don't do anything. This pattern is common in cardiogenic shock and will disappear as Mr. Callan's condition improves.
b) Check the position of the EKG electrodes. They may not be properly secured.
c) Inflate the balloon to determine PCW pressure.
d) Call the doctor immediately to reposition the catheter.

5. Egophony and pectoriloquy are abnormal chest sounds heard in:
a) Cor pulmonale
b) Pulmonary infarction

c) Patients on respirators
d) Pleural effusion
e) All the above

6. Which of the following signs are present in increased intracranial pressure?
a) Shock
b) Bradycardia and widening pulse pressure
c) Hypothermia
d) Pupillary constriction

7. Frank Ritter, 45, is brought to the emergency department in a coma. What should his initial treatment include?
a) I.V. hypertonic glucose
b) Nasal oxygen at 2 to 4 liters
c) A narcotic antagonist (Narcan) for respiratory depression
d) All the above

8. Excessive nitrogen intake or accumulation of nitrogenous body wastes; sepsis; fluid and electrolyte imbalances—what do the above conditions have in common?
a) All may cause blood ammonia levels to rise, leading to hepatic encephalopathy.
b) All may cause rapid and massive liver necrosis, leading to hepatic coma.
c) All may cause cirrhosis in the presence of alcohol.
d) All impede blood flow into the liver, resulting in portal hypertension.

9. Mrs. D'Onofrio, a patient in hepatic failure, has been vomiting lately and has developed signs of metabolic alkalosis and hypokalemia. You know that these conditions increase Mrs. D'Onofrio's risk of falling into hepatic coma. Which of the following would *not* be part of Mrs. D'Onofrio's treatment?
a) Administration of a diuretic
b) Administration of a potassium supplement
c) Measures to prevent nausea, vomiting, diarrhea
d) All the above

(Answers on page 183)

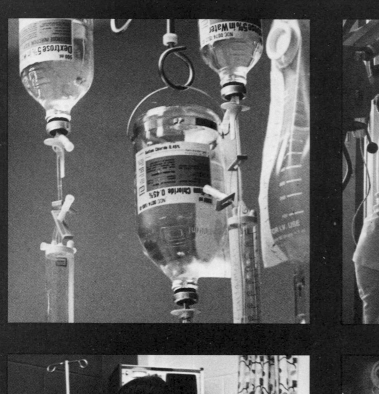

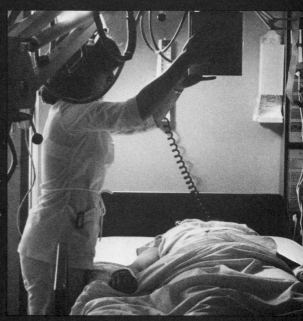

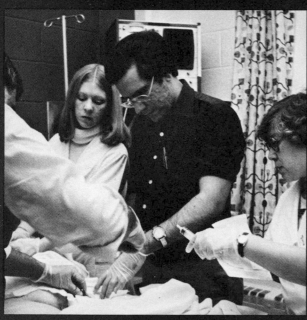

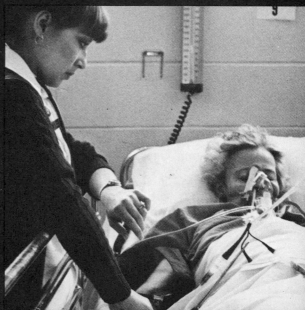

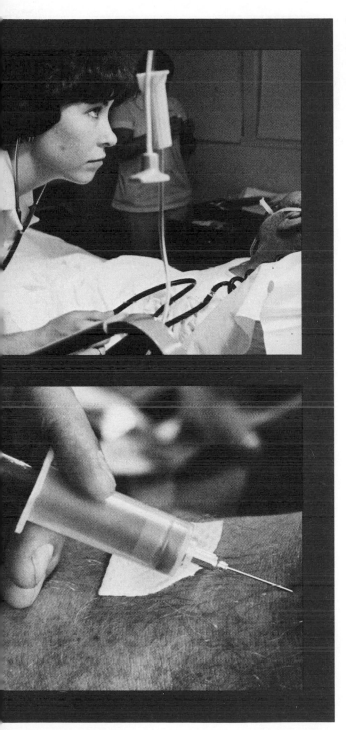

MANAGING SPECIAL PROBLEMS

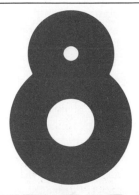

MULTIPLE TRAUMA
Planning the priorities

BY MARILEE MOLYNEUX LUICK, RN

A 38-YEAR-OLD FIREMAN looking for a child's puppy fell through the burning floor of a smoke-filled house....a 56-year-old diabetic with chronic obstructive pulmonary disease and a pacemaker had a massive anterior wall myocardial infarction...a 22-year-old drug dealer was brutally beaten (with a baseball bat and a machete) by two of his customers for selling "bad dope."

These three patients had quite different injuries. Suppose the emergency department called to announce that any one of them was being admitted to your unit. Would you know how to plan for his admission...how to order priorities for his care...how to proceed with his care? In short, would you know what to do? Where to begin?

First, don't panic!
Before such a patient arrives, try to get your own anxieties under control. Just looking at a seriously injured patient can be traumatic even to a seasoned nurse. Remember that the patient is likely to be fully conscious and already emotionally overwhelmed by the disaster that has overtaken him. Avoid adding to his anxieties by looking nervous, shocked, or un-

prepared to give him competent nursing care.

Be better prepared by following a preset routine. A simple alphabetical guide will help you to set your nursing priorities correctly. Simply begin at the beginning...with the letter "A."

A is for airway

An open, patent airway is always your first priority. If the patient is unconscious, check to see if his tongue occludes the airway. Never place a pillow under the head of an unconscious patient unless you have guaranteed an open airway.

If the patient is not breathing, provide artificial ventilation. Even if the patient comes to your unit already intubated, you must still assess for even, bilateral chest excursions and auscultate for bilateral breath sounds. When you admit a patient with multiple-system failure or multiple trauma, carefully evaluate and record baseline breath sounds. Anyone with multiple trauma is especially vulnerable to respiratory insufficiency or ARDS (adult respiratory distress syndrome). If he has had an emergency tracheostomy, watch for bleeding around the stoma, bloody secretions from suctioning, and for gradual swelling of the neck, which could indicate occult hemorrhage or subcutaneous emphysema.

Next, draw a blood sample for arterial blood gases to establish a baseline for oxygen therapy. Every patient with multiple injuries needs supplementary oxygen because of the blood loss and extreme physiologic stress. In fact, the conscious, multiple-trauma victim should be hyperventilating, an emotional and physiologic compensatory mechanism. If he isn't, check for neurologic involvement.

The patient with multiple trauma is likely to be agitated and may try to pull out his airway. Watch for this and prevent it. Consider that he may be just trying to talk. You can help a lot by talking to him while you give him care. Tell him what you're going to do before touching him. Don't forget—even the unconscious patient needs to know what's going on.

Don't be distracted by the obvious. Blood, burns, and mangled joints are dramatic and compel your attention. But don't let them distract you from your first priority, maintaining respiration. The very best wound care won't help if the patient can't breathe. Be especially alert for respiratory distress in any patient who was in a smoky fire, inhaled chemical irritants, or has upper body burns. Breathing in smoke and extremely

MULTIPLE TRAUMA SHEET

Each emergency room should adopt a trauma sheet to standardize assessment and treatment. When completed, the sheet becomes part of the patient's medical record. Typically, a trauma sheet contains the following:

Name_____

Age and sex_____

Approximate weight and height_____

Date and time of admission_____

ASSESSMENT

History of trauma (time, events, weapons, etc.)

Pertinent medical history (allergies, medication taken, chronic diseases, disabilities)

Treatment in progress on admission (check each)

☐ CPR ☐ cardiac monitor
☐ airway ☐ pressure dressings
  (oral or nasal) ☐ back boards
☐ intubation ☐ splints
☐ I.V. therapy ☐ other (explain)

Airway patency

Skin color

Blood pressure (compare to patient's normal B.P.)

Pulse: apical, radial, regular, other

Respiration (regular, tachypneic, apneic)

Breath sounds: left, right (present, diminished, absent) rhonchi, rales

Apparent or possible head injury

Level of consciousness Pain response

☐ alert ☐ appropriate
☐ lethargic ☐ decorticate
☐ stuporous ☐ decerebrate
☐ unconscious ☐ none
☐ other (explain)

Pupillary response to light (left, right); size

Apparent bleeding sites

Foreign objects (weapons) still in wound

Apparent fractures, dislocations

TREATMENT

Airway inserted Tracheostomy:
Intubation: trach size
  tube size performed by
  oral
  nasal
  performed by

Diagnostic tests

☐ complete blood count ☐ SMA$_6$
☐ prothrombin time ☐ SMA$_{12}$
☐ partial thromboplastin time ☐ urinalysis
☐ electrocardiogram ☐ electrolytes
☐ X-ray (kind) ☐ BUN
☐ blood type and match ☐ creatinine

Fluid therapy
  venipuncture or cutdown solutions
  sites amount

Central venous pressure line inserted
  initial reading

Foley catheter inserted (with Urimeter)
  initial amount obtained
  color
  character

Peritoneal lavage:
  intake solution and amount
  output (color, character, amount)

Splints applied

Medications administered

Other

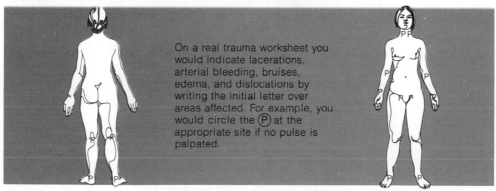

On a real trauma worksheet you would indicate lacerations, arterial bleeding, bruises, edema, and dislocations by writing the initial letter over areas affected. For example, you would circle the (P) at the appropriate site if no pulse is palpated.

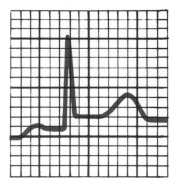

Pericardiocentesis
Pericardiocentesis is needle
aspiration of the pericardial
cavity. It's used to find the
cause of cardiac tamponade
and to relieve it. This procedure
is usually done with the patient
positioned in bed at a 45°
angle. A precordial lead of the
EKG is attached to the
aspirating needle with an alliga-
tor clamp. When the needle
touches the myocardium, you'll
see an S-T segment elevation on
the EKG, as shown above.
   Monitor the patient's blood
pressure during and after this
procedure, and check his
EKG for arrhythmias. Also, keep
an emergency cart with a
defibrillator at the bedside
throughout.

hot air can cause latent laryngeal edema, thermal airway burns,
pneumonitis, and pneumonia.

A patient who has suffered chest trauma usually needs more
than an open airway for oxygenation. He'll probably come to
your unit already intubated, especially if the emergency department staff recognized a flail chest. This kind of patient
may be controlled by mechanical ventilation using positive end
expiratory pressure.

Be ready to manage chest tubes. They're commonly used
with chest injuries that produce hemothorax or pneumothorax. Once in a while, a confused patient will pull out his
chest tube. If this happens, press his gown or sheet against
the opening until you can apply a Vaseline gauze dressing.
Then, call the doctor. When monitoring chest tubes, watch for
subcutaneous emphysema around the insertion site, bloody
drainage of 300 to 500 ml in the first few hours, or a sudden
increase in drainage flow more than 200 ml/hour. Report any
of these immediately. Be careful to maintain patency of the
chest tube. A clogged chest tube can result in tension pneumothorax. If you suspect cardiac tamponade (high CVP, diminished breath sounds, low B.P., paradoxical pulses, jugular
neck-vein distention), notify the doctor immediately. The patient needs an immediate pericardial tap to relieve the pressure.
While assisting the doctor during the procedure, monitor the
EKG to recognize entrance of the needle into the pericardial
sac (usually by S-T elevation) and watch for cardiac arrhythmias. This procedure is dangerous and can be lethal. Usually,
the patient is taken to the O.R. for thoracotomy and insertion
of chest tubes.

A special caution about suctioning: Don't forget to use perfect sterile technique when suctioning to maintain an open
airway. The patient with multiple problems is inevitably vulnerable to infection. As you know, there are bacteria floating
around even the best critical care units.

Report any new sign of respiratory distress. Remember,
dyspnea itself is not solely a symptom of respiratory pathology.
It's also a sign of possible neurologic dysfunction or circulatory imbalance (overload or hypovolemia).

B is for bleeding
After you have established respiratory stability, your next
priority is to recognize bleeding and fluid loss to prevent

DO'S AND DON'TS FOR USING M.A.S.T. EFFECTIVELY

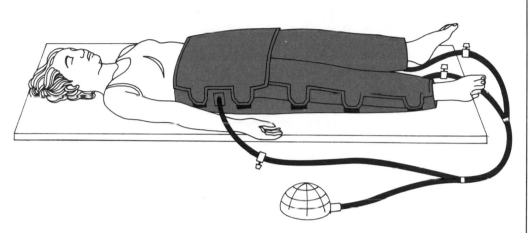

MAST (Medical Anti-Shock Trousers) counteracts bleeding and hypovolemia by slowing or stopping arterial bleeding; by forcing any available blood from the lower body to the heart, brain, and any other vital organ in the upper body; and by preventing return of the available circulating blood volume to the lower extremities.
Do's:
• While patient is wearing MAST: monitor vital signs, blood pressure, apical and radial pulse rate, and respirations; check extremities for pedal pulses, color, warmth, and numbness; and make sure MAST is not too constricting.

• Take MAST off only when: a doctor is present; fluids are available for transfusion; and anesthesia and surgical teams are ready for the patient.
• To clean: Wash with warm soap and water; or air dry and store.
Don'ts:
• Don't apply MAST if: positions or wounds show or suggest intrathoracic or intracranial major vascular injury; patient has open-extremity bleeding, pulmonary edema, or trauma above the level of MAST application.
• When cleaning, don't autoclave or clean with solvents.

shock. Of course, by the time a patient has been transferred from the emergency department to your unit, any overt bleeding will already have been treated. He should have at least one peripheral line and, preferably, a Swan-Ganz or CVP line to guide fluid amount and effect. Watch vital signs even if the patient looks stable. Just because vital signs were taken only 10 minutes before doesn't mean they are still the same. Obtain and record your own baseline readings.

Just moving a multiply injured patient unnecessarily can aggravate or provoke hemorrhage. This doesn't mean you can't carefully examine your new patient. Indeed, you should. If possible—but always carefully—roll the patient over to examine his back only if it has been determined that no cervical spine injury exists. In the frantic pace of the emergency de-

The chest-tube connection

Patients with chest-tube drainage need special care.
• Carefully position the patient.
• Give regular coughing and deep-breathing exercises.
• Make sure that tubing cannot be pulled out, and that it is not kinked or curled.
• Check the amount, color, and consistency of fluid drainage at least hourly for the first 24 hours.
• Check the drainage system. In a bottle setup, the liquid in the glass pipette should rise during inspiration and fall during expiration. In the Pleurevac the liquid should rise on the right side of the chamber and fall on the left side.
• Watch for large amounts of bubbling in the water-seal chamber. A great deal of bubbling may indicate an air leak in the tubing. Check for leakage by clamping the tubing, starting from the top of the drainage tubing and running down to the entry port of the system. Do not keep tubing clamped too long.
• If the drainage system includes suction, check the liquid level in the suction-control chamber during your shift. If the liquid drops below the ordered amount, add enough to maintain the desired level of suction.
• Make sure you can measure the drainage in the bottle system. If the bottle is not precalibrated, get measuring information from the supply personnel so you can calibrate the bottle with tape.
• Always keep drainage bottles or Pleur-evac below the level of the patient's chest.
• Milk and strip chest tubes regularly.
• If a chest tube falls out, occlude the wound immediately with sterile Vaseline gauze and call for help.

partment, some potentially serious things can be overlooked in the supine patient. Some surprising items I have found by such examinations have included: glass fragments, a broken knife imbedded in a buttock, a spent rifle cartridge, and teeth and dentures.

Keep in mind that "normal" vital signs in a single assessment do not indicate stability. A person can lose 20% of blood volume before his blood pressure drops. A young patient, especially, can (by peripheral vasoconstriction) temporarily maintain his blood pressure at an acceptable level despite dangerous blood loss. In such a patient, you might not hear Korotkoff's sounds, but you could get a palpable blood pressure of 100. When in doubt, use a Doppler manometer to confirm your blood pressure reading.

Don't overlook the fact that a profusely bleeding patient is also "bleeding" oxygen. He'll be tachypneic and may develop cardiac arrest from hypoxia if he doesn't get prompt blood replacement and oxygen. Before admission to your unit, the E.D. should have obtained a type and crossmatch along with a CBC, chemistry profile, prothrombin time and partial prothrombin time, followed by blood replacement as needed. If the blood the patient receives isn't warmed first, every unit of blood can lower the patient's body temperature by 1° C. If the patient needs multiple units of blood, he'll also need fresh frozen plasma, platelets, packed RBCs, and clotting factors.

In most hospitals, albumin is out of favor for treating hypovolemia because of its tendency to produce pulmonary fluid overload. Solutions containing dextran are also out of favor. Dextran makes the platelets "slippery," increasing the potential for bleeding. If you're dealing with a burn victim, you'll have to correct hemoconcentration, not hypovolemia. A burn victim usually doesn't need blood. He usually does need massive fluid replacement, precisely measured and carefully monitored.

A Swan-Ganz pulmonary artery line offers the most accurate way to measure the effects of fluid therapy as it reflects left heart function. A pulmonary wedge pressure (PWP) higher than 15 indicates developing cardiac overload. If you use a CVP line, its readings reflect a change in the ability of the right ventricle to accept fluid. When volume replacement fails to raise an initially low CVP reading, consider this a sign of

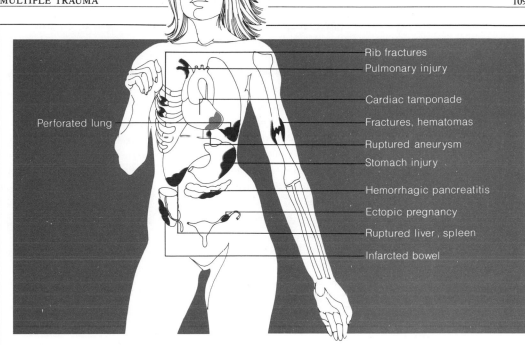

Perforated lung

Rib fractures
Pulmonary injury

Cardiac tamponade

Fractures, hematomas

Ruptured aneurysm

Stomach injury

Hemorrhagic pancreatitis

Ectopic pregnancy

Ruptured liver, spleen

Infarcted bowel

continuous fluid loss.

Be constantly alert for signs of occult bleeding. Common sites of such bleeding include the chest, the abdomen, and a fractured pelvis or femur (see illustration above). Use a tape measure to assess occult bleeding. Mark the placement of the tape measure, so that the same diameter is used consistently to accurately reflect size changes. Increased diameter of a limb, the abdomen, or pelvis often points to blood or plasma seepage into these tissues. As much as 2000 ml can seep into the thigh; 4000 ml into the pelvis and abdomen; and 3000 ml into the thorax. A patient with such blood loss will show classic signs of hypovolemic shock (rapid pulse and respirations, falling blood pressure, restlessness, falling urinary output, and cold clammy skin), but you won't see any blood. Occasionally you can detect occult abdominal hemorrhage by finding a retroperitoneal hematoma. Be aware that retroperitoneal bleeding may not result in abdominal tenderness. Symptoms may include numbness and pain in a lower extremity as the result of compressing the lateral femoral cutaneous nerve, which is in the region of L1 to L3,. Expect this if you know your patient has renal injuries or a fractured pelvis.

Hidden threat
With multiple-trauma patients, you must be alert to signs of occult bleeding. This illustration shows the usual sites of such bleeding, along with the probable causes.

Shock syndromes likely

The patient with multiple trauma or multiple-system failure is predisposed to almost all "shock syndromes."

Of course, hypovolemic shock is the most common form. The patient with major hemorrhage almost always shows the classic signs of hypovolemia. A patient with acute dehydration and severe burns can develop hypovolemic shock.

Septic shock is a potentially lethal complication you always want to prevent, or at least recognize early. Never let your haste to give complicated care as efficiently as possible distract you from strict aseptic technique when using suction, urinary catheters, I.V. equipment, and endotracheal tubes, and when applying dressings. All of these can readily serve as channels of infection.

Because the skin serves as the body's first line of defense, patients with large areas of broken skin are special candidates for sepsis. Burn victims are especially so and need meticulous isolation techniques to prevent it.

Watch for DIC (disseminated intravascular coagulation). Some experts consider it a form of septic shock. Report any serosanguineous oozing from puncture sites, body orifices, hematuria, hematemesis, or other signs of this mysterious bleeding/clotting phenomenon as soon as possible (see also Chapter 13).

Watch for cardiogenic shock, a potential complication in patients with multiple problems, especially if they have a cardiac history, acute myocardial infarction, or any injury to the heart. In such patients, fluid overload can lead to pump failure. Both cardiogenic shock and fluid overload can lead to adult respiratory distress syndrome (ARDS) if allowed to persist.

Don't overlook the possibility of anaphylactic shock. Watch for the subtle signs of anaphylaxis: low-grade temperature, irritability, dull back pain, increased respiratory rate, and pruritus. Report and treat them before the obvious signs of full-blown anaphylactic shock (laryngeal edema and cardiovascular collapse) develop. Anaphylaxis is a special problem in critically ill patients. Their illnesses are complex, and so is their treatment. Almost all of them need simultaneous treatment with fluid replacement, blood, and large doses and combinations of multiple pharmacologic agents (especially antibiotics, steroids, analgesics, and cardiovascular drugs). So make it your business to know these agents' incompatibilities, contraindi-

COPING WITH COMPLICATIONS

Sepsis and pulmonary embolism are a constant threat to the multiple trauma patient. You can play a big part in recognizing these complications early, and in preventing them:
- Always maintain sterile technique. Don't forget to wash hands often.
- Keep visitors and staff with colds or other infections off the unit.
- Check lab reports, especially for white count.
- Note character of patient's sputum and urine. Obtain cultures when indicated.
- Turn patient frequently. Apply heel pads or sheepskin when needed.

SEPSIS AND SEPTIC SHOCK
Sepsis can strike any multiple trauma patient and may lead to septic shock, which has two phases. In warm shock the patient is alert and has a good urinary flow and a pink flush This phase is followed by cold shock, characterized by cold and clammy skin, pallor, hypotension, and decreased circulation.

Since septic shock can progress rapidly to death (survival rate is less than 30%), don't wait for confirming or culture reports before beginning treatment. Besides giving massive doses of I.V. antibiotics, treatment is primarily supportive.

PULMONARY EMBOLISM
Multiple trauma patients are also especially prone to pulmonary embolism. It usually originates from the deep veins in the legs. Observe these patients' calves for tenderness, increased diameter, warm spots, and erythema. Encourage patients to move their legs and wiggle their toes, and warn them not to cross their legs. For patients unable to move, do passive and active ROM exercises, change their positions frequently, and apply anti-emboli T.E.D. stockings or Ace bandages, if needed. Regularly do chest physiotherapy to mobilize secretions and to facilitate breathing and circulation.

cations, and side effects. Mix nothing together until you have verified what the combined effect will be.

C is for consciousness

Your continuing assessment of your patient's level of consciousness serves as an index of adequate cerebral ventilation and perfusion. Always assume that the critically ill patient whose responses seem confused or inappropriate has some physiologic imbalance before you blame his behavior on emotional problems. Don't forget that the sensory deprivations imposed by treatment in a critical care unit can confuse anyone (including some nurses). So, provide reinforcements for your patient's time and place orientation (clocks, calendars, radios, and pictures of loved ones).

In determining level of consciousness, define it in terms accepted and understood by your institution and other members of the staff. Report decorticate and decerebrate responses as soon as they appear. Remember that the patient need not have a head injury to show inappropriate neurologic response. A metabolic failure that causes inadequate ventilation or perfusion will produce cerebral edema and intracranial pressure. But if your patient has neurologic symptoms and is hypotensive, look for an extracranial cause; intracranial bleeding does not produce hypovolemic shock except in infants. Assess pupil reactivity periodically to determine progression of neurologic involvement and effectiveness of treatment. A patient in deep metabolic coma tends to have normal pupillary responses; conversely, an alert, head-injured patient tends to have strongly pathologic pupillary responses.

Remember the special risk of infection when the integrity of the cerebrospinal system has been broached. The risk of infection is the same whether the spinal fluid was invaded through a meningeal tear, or by the insertion of a subarachnoid screw or intraventricular catheter for ICP monitoring. In either case, the patient needs special safeguards against infection.

D is for digestion

Patients with multiple problems should receive nothing by mouth until their condition has been carefully identified and stabilized. They usually need a nasogastric tube to aspirate stomach contents, decompress the stomach, and disclose any bleeding. If unconscious, they usually need intubation to guarantee a patent airway before you pass a nasogastric tube.

Because patients with multiple problems are in stressful states producing high-energy expenditure, they need extra calories to maintain a positive nitrogen balance. They must be specially fed, starting almost immediately after admission. The old routine of 1000 ml of 5% dextrose in water every 8 hours provides only 500 calories in 24 hours—or the equivalent of one piece of apple pie. For adequate nutrition, these patients need hyperalimentation parenterally or via tube feedings. Hyperalimentation provides the calories and nutrients they need to satisfy their energy requirements for recovery.

Prevent stress ulcers. They're a common phenomenon in critically ill patients—especially those on respirators and those who receive nothing by mouth. Such ulcers are likely to cause gastric bleeding from hyperacidity. Tube feedings every 2 to 4 hours, especially with an antacid, help prevent them.

Inspect the patient's abdomen for scars and injuries. Report their configuration and size. If you notice gradual expansion in girth, think of hemorrhage or organic enlargement (especially of the liver). Report any abdominal pain. Of course, you can't relieve such pain with medication until you know what's causing it. Also evaluate the location, intensity, and radiation of the pain. To find out what's causing abdominal pain, first check the patient's history and physical examination for clues (that may be confirmed by an X-ray flat plate of the abdomen). Next auscultate bowel sounds. Are they regular and frequent? If not, consider ileus. Does the patient in whom you find edema of the right upper quadrant complain of right-sided tenderness? Consider liver damage. Do you find an elevated white blood count, left flank pain, and upper quadrant pain radiating to the left shoulder (Kehr's signs)? Consider splenic laceration or rupture. Be prepared to assist with a paracentesis (to remove excess fluid and for diagnostic evaluation) and peritoneal lavage (to rule out bleeding). In either case, prepare your patient for the procedure by letting him know exactly what to expect.

E is for excretion

Although the trend is to avoid catheters because of the risk of infection, critically ill patients with multiple problems almost always need a Foley catheter. An indwelling catheter allows continuous readings of urine output—an index of kidney function and of the effect of fluid therapy and replacement. In adults, a safe output is greater than 50 ml/hr. Also measure specific gravity to determine the concentration of urine.

Many of the drugs critically ill patients receive (such as large doses of antibiotics) are nephrotoxic and ototoxic. Monitor drug effects carefully. Follow renal function studies including BUN and creatinine; and, in your patients who are already hypotensive, remember to check for an adequate fluid replacement before giving a vasoconstricting drug. Otherwise, acute tubule necrosis can result.

Also analyze urine output for: concentration (a sign of dehydration); purulent drainage (a sign of infection, sometimes the result of instrumentation); and hematuria (which may not be directly related to renal function). Hematuria occurs in 85% to 90% of all multiple-trauma victims, probably due to the great force or pressure exerted on body tissues during trauma. Remember that DIC also produces hematuria; so does overdosage with anticoagulants.

Watch urinary output carefully and report changes in it promptly. Especially report decreasing output. Don't wait until kidney output fails completely. If renal failure does occur, treatment usually consists of fluid challenges, diuretics, peritoneal dialysis, and hemodialysis.

The fat of the matter

Fat embolism is an ever-present danger after multiple trauma, especially after multiple fractures. Why? One theory holds that catecholamines released as part of the stress response mobilize fatty acids, which alter fat emulsion and make fat embolism possible. Also, fractures, especially of the long bones, release fat droplets from the marrow, which may lodge in the lungs or even the brain.

Fat embolism often occurs within 24 hours after a trauma, but may be delayed up to 72 hours. Unlike shock, it usually doesn't develop during the first 12 hours after the trauma. What are the signs of fat embolism? Look for apprehension, mild agitation, sweating, fever, tachycardia, pallor, shortness of breath, disturbances in consciousness, tissue hypoxia, and cyanosis.

The most distinctive sign, though, is a rash on the chest and shoulders, which may extend to the axillae, flanks, soft palate mucosa, and the conjunctiva.

If you suspect fat embolism, immediately immobilize the patient and call the doctor. Stay with the patient to give him reassurance and support. Have the patient breathe deeply. Give oxygen via cannula or mask. When necessary, mechanical ventilation or support with PEEP can maintain oxygenation.

The doctor may order corticosteroids, I.V. dextrose and water with ethanol, and heparin. He may also order a diuretic such as furosemide (Lasix) to reduce interstitial edema.

F is for fractures

This final step applies to the patient with multiple trauma (who almost invariably has fractures). If he comes to your unit before surgery, keep splints and backboards in place. Inspect splinted areas carefully for bleeding, especially in fractures located near major vessels. Palpate pulses distal to the fracture to rule out arterial insufficiency. Watch for the "5 Ps" that point to arterial insufficiency . . .

- Pulses decreased or absent
- Pallor
- Paresthesias
- Pain
- Paralysis

If the patient has a closed fracture of the pelvis, hip, or femur, take girth measurements to rule out occult bleeding. If he has an open fracture, clean it carefully with sterile normal saline. Keep it covered with an iodine dressing until surgery.

Occasionally, you'll see a patient in whom soft tissue and bone trauma has created a traumatic A-V fistula. In such a patient, arterial circulation is prematurely shunted back into the venous system around the trauma site. Identify a traumatic A-V fistula by palpating a thrill and hearing a bruit on auscultation over the trauma site. Premature venous return increases cardiac output, possibly overloading the right heart to the point of high-output cardiac failure. Check carefully for traumatic fistula because of these severe consequences.

You're well aware that fat emboli of long-bone fractures are a potentially fatal complication. Characteristically, fat emboli produce agitation, confusion, a body rash (especially in the groin, axilla, and sclerae), and, eventually, severe respiratory distress. Know what you can do to prevent fat emboli (see margin, page 113).

The alphabetical approach to care for multiple disease and trauma was designed to serve as a guide to emergency assessment and treatment. It's a systematic way of identifying and keeping track of all a patient's injuries and should be routine nursing practice. It's just as useful for keeping your priorities in order after a patient reaches the critical care unit or the regular medical-surgical unit. If you use this guide consistently, you're sure to grow more competent and, consequently, feel more confident when caring for patients who are critically ill.

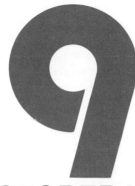

POSTOPERATIVE RECOVERY
Monitoring for physiologic equilibrium

BY THERESA CROUSHORE, RN

IT'S SATURDAY NIGHT on the medical/surgical floor. You're expecting a patient who just had an emergency cholecystectomy, and he's coming directly from the O.R. Are you prepared to give him the special care he needs during his recovery from anesthesia? Do you know how often to check vital signs...how to know when his condition is stable...how to recognize abnormal drainage? This chapter will tell you how.

A critical time

Recovery from anesthesia is the time of physiologic disequilibrium. It's a critical time when many postoperative complications are possible. For example, shock and anoxemia due to respiratory difficulties are common, as you know. To deal with them promptly and prevent them from becoming catastrophic, you must closely monitor postoperative patients until the major effects of anesthetic and adjunctive drugs have dissipated; that is, until they're reasonably conscious and in stable condition.

Immediate postanesthetic assessment and care rely heavily on skilled nursing observations. Knowing something about anesthetic agents and the drugs and the equipment commonly

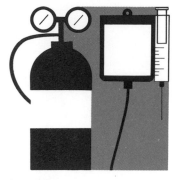

As surgery goes on
Preparations for postop care
should begin while the patient is
in surgery. Here are some tips to
help you get ready.
• Make sure the patient's bed is
secured and made. Place the
bedding properly but don't tuck it
in. Protect the mattress and
pillows from emesis or drainage
as necessary. In all cases, you'll
want to place side rails on the
bed to prevent the patient from
falling out. In other cases, you'll
need to put a board under the
mattress for additional support.
Then adjust the height of the bed
so it matches the height of the
stretcher used to return the
patient to his room.
• Set a comfortable room
temperature.
• Anticipate what equipment to
have on hand and make sure it
works. What you'll need will
depend on the kind of surgery
involved, the kind of anesthetic
used, and the position the patient
will assume.
• Have suction equipment, a
Gomco machine, oxygen, and/or
a tracheostomy tray available as
needed. For example, the patient
returning from abdominal surgery
may have an nasogastric tube in
place. Make sure the Gomco
machine works and is in
position.

used in the operating room does help you to analyze and
predict patient responses. But your most reliable information
about recovery from anesthesia takes highly developed skills
in routine observation and assessment.

To keep up with the potentially rapid changes during this
critical time, your baseline assessment must be accurate,
complete, and fast. And you must record your assessment
accurately so that nurses who continue his care will have a
reference point from which to proceed. This can be a lot less
difficult if you have a workable system for gathering information in an organized way, and use it consistently. A simple
mnemonic can help you to remember one routine for systematic assessment: Could an RN Want to GUess what is
GoIng on? Surely, you don't want to guess. You can be
certain about the patient's condition if you check systems in
this order: Circulatory, Respiratory, Neurologic, Wound,
GenitoUrinary, and GastroIntestinal.

Let's see how such assessment works in a typical patient.
Mr. Scott, a 45-year-old butcher, came to our unit directly
from the O.R. after a cholecystectomy under general anesthesia. While guiding the stretcher to his room, I began his
baseline assessment. I noticed his skin was pink, warm, and
dry. His airway was patent; his respirations were slow, even,
deep, and effective. While helping Mr. Scott into his bed, I
noticed that his muscular coordination was intact, but fine
coordination was still depressed. As soon as he was settled in
his bed, I checked his blood pressure and apical and radial
pulses. His cardiopulmonary functions had remained stable
during the transfer. His surgical dressings were dry and intact
with no through drainage. His abdomen was flat. I.V. fluids
were infusing well. His nasogastric tube was patent, with
clear, watery reflux. Mr. Scott greeted his wife with a drowsy
nod as I checked his temperature and connected his drainage
tubes to the proper collection devices.

With just this thumbnail assessment, and with information
from the O.R. nurse, I knew that Mr. Scott was reacting
normally for his stage of recovery — his cardiopulmonary
status was good, his wound site was intact, and he had
remained stable during the transfer. I could continue more
detailed assessment by organ system.

Let's look at the system-by-system assessment in more
detail.

Circulatory assessment

To determine the patient's circulatory status, you must frequently check blood pressure and pulses. These are the most important criteria for determining circulatory status. Note the rate, rhythm, and character of the apical and radial pulses and check for presence of peripheral arterial pulses. When auscultating an apical pulse, be sure to listen for *one minute*, at least. When evaluating circulatory signs, remember that they vary a great deal. They vary normally with age and sex. They also vary with medications, hemodynamic changes, pain, fever, emotional state, positioning, and the presence of cardiopulmonary disease.

Also, notice the effect of circulation on interrelating systems. For example, is inadequate perfusion affecting the kidneys (low output) or the brain (restlessness, confusion)? Both of these effects are common immediately postanesthesia. So are cardiac arrhythmias. Watch carefully for arrhythmias; recognizing them promptly and managing them correctly can prevent lasting damage. (Chronic arrhythmias need not be treated at this time unless they are hazardous.) Make it your business to know the patient's cardiac history. It will help you evaluate his circulatory status correctly.

Expect and look for signs of compensation — a physiologic adjustment to surgical trauma. Patients who've undergone major thoracic or abdominal surgery readily display systemic signs of compensation. For example, their body temperature normally rises to 99.3° F. (37.7° C.) for 24 to 48 hours after surgery. Also, their extremities may differ markedly from the central body in color and temperature. They may look flushed and have a warm face and torso but cool, pale arms and legs. Watch for this situation. It points to early shock with compensation. Many patients returning from surgery feel cold and benefit from a few *warmed* blankets. Remember to remove extra blankets when they've recovered from anesthesia.

Don't forget: A reliable source of information about circulatory status is the appearance of the blood itself. When restarting an I.V., or giving an injection, notice the color, consistency, and clotting ability of the blood. Many lab tests have confirmed an astute nurse's observation of hemodilution: "When I restarted the I.V., I noticed the patient's blood looked watery and pale."

Respiratory assessment

During respiratory assessment, you must evaluate airway patency, chest symmetry, depth, rate, and character of the respirations, and the effort needed to elicit them. Also, watch the effects of deep-breathing and coughing exercises, and gauge the amount of air actually moved in and out of the lungs. Notice and record the character of any sputum or mucus. Mucus from the trachea or throat usually looks watery and colorless; sputum from the bronchi or lungs looks thick and yellow-tinged; sputum that's frothy and white suggests congestive heart failure or pulmonary edema; greenish sputum suggests pneumonia.

When evaluating respirations, ask yourself: *Are the patient's respirations effective?* Notice the patient's circumstances (whether he's receiving oxygen; what position he's in; and what are his emotional and psychologic states?) and do what you can to continue them. If his respirations are not effective, why not? Is he in pain, or is his airway obstructed by mucus, sputum, or tubing (such as a nasogastric tube)? You'll need to suction the recovering patient periodically because he can't mobilize the secretions himself. What position is he in? The best position for the postanesthetic patient is supine with his head turned to one side *(but only if the patient is constantly attended)*. However, if the patient might be alone for any time, position him on his side with his head tilted back and supported. These positions, which allow the most lung expansion and the greatest airway patency, prevent aspiration of emesis. If the patient has received spinal anesthesia, be sure to keep the bed flat—although you may place a pillow under his head.

Remember that after prolonged anesthesia or use of muscle-relaxing drugs such as curare, many patients have *no muscular control* during recovery. Paralyzed laryngotracheal muscles create difficulty with breathing: choking, noisy and irregular respirations. But, remember that some patients with airway obstruction make no telltale sounds. So make sure you periodically check the airway for patency, and maintain head tilt. If you *do* notice difficulty in breathing, check the airway. Use the triple airway maneuver, or jaw thrust, to hold the patient's tongue forward to open the air passages. You can grasp the tongue more easily with gauze (rather than with a gloved or bare hand). When such maneuvers become

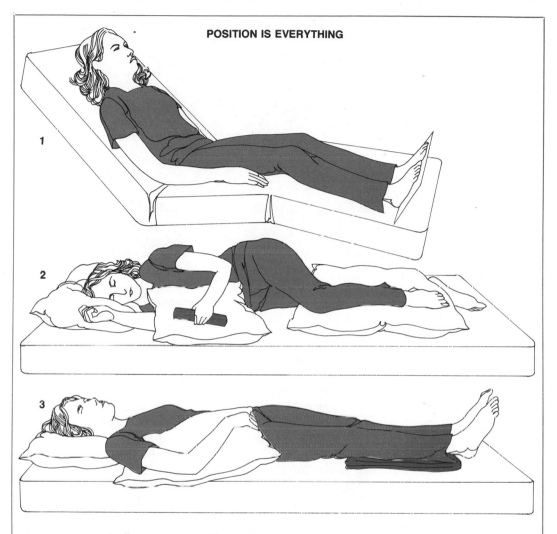

POSITION IS EVERYTHING

The position of a patient recovering from surgery is all-important. Place the patient in a semi-Fowler's position to prevent her tongue from occluding her airway and prevent aspiration of any regurgitated liquids that are pooled in her pharynx (Fig. 1). Or place the patient in a lateral position with her head tilted back and down, her face toward the pillow, so that secretions can drain outside her mouth or pool inside her cheeks where they can be suctioned safely (Fig. 2).

Do not use the supine position unless you are constantly monitoring the patient or you have turned the patient's head toward the pillow (Fig. 3).

Positioning the patient correctly for postop recovery serves several purposes:
- It facilitates drainage of respiratory and gastric secretions.
- It prevents aspiration of these secretions or of emesis.
- It helps maintain an adequate airway and facilitates breathing.
- It prevents spinal headache.
- It promotes patient comfort.

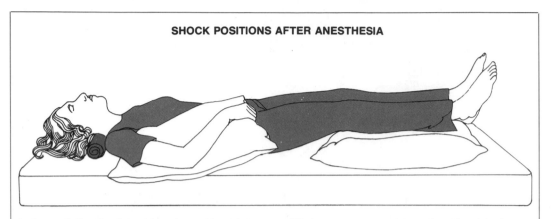

SHOCK POSITIONS AFTER ANESTHESIA

In the past, the shock position of choice was the Trendelenburg — the patient lying supine with the lower end of her body elevated above her head. This was thought to increase venous return and improve cerebral blood flow. In fact, this position doesn't do either.

Nowadays, a modified Trendelenburg position is preferred. Elevate the patient's legs just enough to create a gradual downward slope toward her upper torso. This will facilitate the drainage of secretions.

CAUTION: Never place a patient who's had spinal anesthesia or a craniotomy in a Trendelenburg position, modified or otherwise. This position can paralyze the diaphragm and increase intracranial edema and pressure. Have such a patient lie flat, elevate her head 30°, and place a plump pillow under each of her arms and legs.

necessary, better insert a plastic or hard-rubber airway.

Next, evaluate respirations. Though spirometers are useful, you really need only your own hand. Cup your hand, palm down, over the patient's nose and mouth, feel the forcefulness of the exhaled breath. Would the exhaled puff you felt fill a sandwich-size Baggie with air? If not, respirations are not yet deep enough. You may then have to assist ventilation with an Ambu bag and mask.

Many things can change the rate and depth of respirations: level of consciousness, insufficient or excessive oxygen, medications, body position, pain, and apprehension. So consider these factors. Evaluate the patient's chest for symmetry. Also notice the abdominal or accessory muscles. If the patient is using these muscles to breathe, he may be developing severe respiratory distress.

Listen for breath sounds. They are decreased or absent when air flow is diminished, or when fluid or tissue separates the air passages from the bell of the stethoscope. So you can expect diminished breath sounds in both pulmonary edema and obesity. Breath sounds may also be absent when the endotracheal (ET) tube obstructs the lungs. This tube may still be in place in the postanesthetic patient. Since the tracheal angle on the right is less acute, the left lung could be occluded if the ET tube is placed too far down the right main stem bronchus. Don't assume that because the patient had undergone surgery with the tube in place that it is still correctly placed. Remember, it's a movable tube and tends to slide even when taped. Use your stethoscope to validate breath sounds in both lungs. When tube position is in doubt, a chest X-ray can determine correct placement. Correctly placed, the tip of the tube is above the carina.

When can you remove the ET tube? Several guidelines help you to know when a patient can resume respiration without help. Generally, you can safely remove the ET tube when...

• The patient can lift his head off the pillow and hold it up for 30 seconds

• The patient is moving adequate air (as evidenced by the Baggie test).

Some nurses mistakenly feel that when a patient is ready to have the ET tube or airway removed, he'll remove it himself. This is unsafe practice. A delirious patient may inadvertently pull at any tube he can. So, don't abdicate your nursing judgment to a partially anesthetized patient. Always make this decision yourself based on information you have about the patient's condition.

Also, listen for coarse rales (the rough, gurgling sound heard over the lungs at the beginning of inspiration). They indicate a need for nasotracheal suctioning of the secretions producing the rales.

Neurologic assessment
To assess neurologic status, you must evaluate the patient's level of consciousness. Anesthetized patients usually return to consciousness in a predictable pattern: muscular irritability, restlessness and delirium, consciousness, the ability to perceive pain and, finally, the ability to perceive pain before the ability to reason and control behavior. However, these stages vary slightly depending on the anesthetic used and on the patient's preoperative condition. Obviously, the patient who is recovering from anesthesia needs repeated orientation and reassurance. Simple explanations and commands are most effective during this time. The ability to follow com-

WHAT YOU SHOULD KNOW ABOUT COMMON ANESTHETIC AGENTS			
ANESTHETIC AGENT	ROUTE AND CHARACTERISTICS	SIDE EFFECTS AND INTERACTIONS	NURSING CONSIDERATIONS
fentanyl with droperidol (Innovar)	• Given I.V. or I.M. • Short-acting combination of narcotic analgesic and major tranquilizer. • Usually given 45 to 60 minutes before surgery, with or without atropine. • Besides anesthesia, produces antiemetic, alpha-adrenergic blocking, and antiarrhythmic effects.	• Hallucinations, depression, unusual drowsiness lasting up to 1 week; bradycardia, circulatory collapse, hypotension, increased pulmonary artery pressure; apnea, laryngospasm, bronchospasm, hypoventilation, rigidity of respiratory muscles; other muscle rigidity. • May be habit-forming. • Potentiates CNS depressants.	• Keep atropine available to treat bradycardia. • Keep CPR and airway intubation equipment, neuromuscular blocker, and narcotic antagonist available to treat respiratory complications. Narcotic antagonist alone is not sufficient to reverse respiratory symptoms. • O₂ is recommended postop. • Check vital signs often. • Reduce doses of CNS depressants by ⅓ to ½ at least 8 hours postanesthesia.
halothane (Fluothane)	• General inhalation anesthetic used with N₂O or muscle relaxant. • Produces rapid and smooth induction.	• Cardiac rate and rhythm changes (bradycardia, nodal rhythm, AV dislocation); decreased cardiac output with resulting hypotension (with high concentrations); ventricular fibrillation (when used with epinephrine and norepinephrine); tachypnea; hepatic dysfunction. • CNS depressants (including alcohol) potentiate halothane effect. • Seldom causes nausea or vomiting; nonirritating to mucous membranes.	• Patient awakes slowly after long procedures on high concentrations. • Check vital signs often. Hyperventilation can rapidly reverse effect. • Keep atropine available to reverse bradycardia. • Record all premedications carefully. • Shivering is common in recovery phase.
ketamine HCl (Ketaject, Ketalar)	• Given I.V. or I.M. • Short-acting nonbarbiturate. • Causes dissociative anesthesia of rapid onset and short duration. • Used in short procedures or for induction with general anesthetic.	• Visual hallucinations, confusion may occur within 24 hours, especially if patient has organic brain syndrome; elevated cerebrospinal fluid pressure; elevated blood pressure; transient respiratory depression. • Does not change pharyngeal-laryngeal reflexes or auditory function.	• Keep side rails up and observe patient closely for 24 hours after anesthesia. • Protect patient from sudden verbal, tactile, or visual stimulation. • Keep CPR equipment with airway available. • Check vital signs often. • Small dose of short-acting barbiturate may be used to reverse emergency reaction. • Recovery time may be prolonged if used with barbiturates or narcotics.

WHAT YOU SHOULD KNOW ABOUT COMMON ANESTHETIC AGENTS

ANESTHETIC AGENT	ROUTE AND CHARACTERISTICS	SIDE EFFECTS AND INTERACTIONS	NURSING CONSIDERATIONS
lidocaine HCl (Xylocaine)	• Local, peripheral, field block, or spinal anesthetic.	• Stimulation, such as laughing, crying, excessive talking; drowsiness; hypotension, bradycardia, cardiac arrest, depressed myocardium and conduction system; respiratory depression or arrest; sweating.	• Keep O$_2$, CPR equipment, and airway available. • Keep vasopressors and volume expanders available to treat hypotension. • Check vital signs often. • Don't use lidocaine with epinephrine for anesthetic block of digits. • Lidocaine with epinephrine is contraindicated in elderly or those with heart disease.
methoxyflurane (Penthrane)	• General inhalation anesthetic. • Often used with N$_2$O, sodium pentothal, or muscle relaxants. • Potent anesthetic; used in short procedures because it's rapidly metabolized.	• Nephrotoxic. • May enhance adverse renal effects of antibiotics (tetracycline, garamycin, tobramycin, kanamycin). • CNS depressants (alcohol) potentiate effect. • Seldom causes nausea, vomiting, or arrhythmias.	• Prolonged postop drowsiness and analgesia are likely. • Check vital signs often. • Hyperventilation can rapidly reverse effect. • Record all premedications carefully.
nitrous oxide (N$_2$O)	• General inhalation anesthetic for rapid induction. • Not a potent anesthetic. Must be administered with O$_2$. • Nonirritating to mucous membrane.	• Arterial hypoxemia. Poor muscle relaxation. • CNS depressants (including alcohol) potentiate N$_2$O effect.	• To prevent diffusion hypoxia, give O$_2$ therapy by nasal prongs or mask. • Check vital signs often. Hyperventilation can rapidly reverse effect. • Record all premedications carefully. • Keep ABG kit available.
thiopental sodium (Pentothal)	• Given I.V. or rectally. • Barbiturate with rapid onset and short duration. • Used in short (15-minute) surgical procedures; for induction with regional or general anesthetic, and with hypnosis.	• Cardiac depression, hypotension, respiratory depression, apnea, laryngeal spasm with cyanosis. • Seldom causes cardiac arrhythmias.	• Check vital signs often; blood pressure may drop rapidly. • Keep CPR and intubation equipment, and tracheostomy tray available. • Maintain adequate postop patient position. • Patient may appear to wake up completely but returns to anesthesia state when undisturbed. • Shivering, coughing, and sneezing are common in recovery phase.

Route side effects

Sometimes the very route by which a regional anesthetic is administered will produce complications or side effects. For example, local anesthetics are often injected into the epidural space — commonly in the lumbar area — within the vertebral canal. The epidural route affords easy administration, minimal trauma to the spinal cord, and widespread sympathetic blockade. And because it does not puncture the dural space, patients seldom suffer a spinal headache. However, because the epidural space is highly vascular, a high dosage may cause systemic toxic effects. So report CNS disturbances, rising blood pressure, and a rapid pulse to the doctor.

When a local anesthetic is injected directly into the cerebral spinal fluid (CSF), it produces sympathetic blockade. Patients who are anesthetized by the *spinal route* may suffer a spinal headache, caused by CSF leaking around the dural puncture site. By sitting up, the patient may reduce CSF pressure. He may even experience diplopia and tinnitus.

You can help. Keep the patient in a horizontal position and, unless contraindicated, keep him well hydrated. Give mild analgesia p.r.n. If the patient's headache is severe, consult with the doctor. He may inject normal saline solution into the epidural space to prevent further CSF leakage.

mands is a good indicator of the neurologic status.

Keep in mind the many factors that can affect the level of consciousness: medications; emotional state; hemodynamics; lack of natural sleep; and electrolyte imbalance. (Watch laboratory reports for electrolyte levels, BUN, CBC, and check intake and output balance record.)

Evaluating pain can be difficult. Body language, such as clenched fists, furrowed brow, and sighing respirations can suggest the presence of pain or an emotional state. So can diaphoresis, rapid pulse, restlessness, or reluctance to move. So watch for these clues. However, until the patient is fully recovered, be especially careful about giving pain medications; you know pain medications interact with and potentiate the residual effects of some anesthetics.

Record the location, type and duration of pain, environmental circumstances, and whether or not the pain is relieved, increased, or decreased by medications, rest, position, exercise, or verbalization. If the patient is conscious, be guided by the patient's own description of the pain. Keep in mind that postoperative pain can have several causes: The dressing may be too bulky, the pain medication may not be strong enough, or the patient may have a tolerance to it. His pain threshold may be low. Or he may simply have *expected* a lot of postoperative pain.

Restlessness and muscle irritability are common after surgery. After anesthesia that includes thiopental sodium (Sodium Pentothal), patients commonly develop the "Pentothal shakes." This is a sign of muscular irritability that closely resembles shivering. It's a transient phenomenon, but one the patient finds distressing. Record among your observations: the patient's muscular coordination, and the time at which motion and sensation return to the anesthetized area. Ability to accurately perceive a pinprick confirms return of sensation.

Remember to consider the patient's emotional status, which you can interpret largely by his behavior. Apathy, anxiety, anger, fear, and tension are common reactions to pain and illness. When evaluating psychologic and neurologic symptoms, validate your findings by comparing them with the staff's or the patient's family's preoperative observations.

Wound assessment

Watch the surgical wound carefully and see it as more than

just a skin incision. After abdominal surgery, the incision extends through skin, fat, fascia, muscle, and peritoneum to a particular organ. Most surgical wounds are clean, closely sutured wounds which heal by first intention. They may or may not have protective sterile dressings; however, most do — at least at first. Expect a small amount of serous drainage from any incision, but remember that some incisions have more or different drainage. So when observing a surgical wound, always notice the amount, color, odor, and consistency of drainage. You can measure the amount of drainage by weighing the dressings or by recording the size of the enlarging circle of drainage. Outline the circle of drainage on the dressing with a marking pen, along with the date and time. Include this information in your notes along with the date and time you observed it. Keep in mind that some patients come from surgery with a Penrose drain in the incision. Such a drain will wet the dressing. Unless you think of a Penrose drain and check the patient's chart for it whenever you see a wet dressing, you might become unduly alarmed (see page 129, *Normal Tube Drainage*).

When evaluating your observations about a surgical wound, ask yourself two key questions: Is there any change in the amount, color, consistency, or odor of the drainage from the incision or tubes? If so, why? For example, if a previously dry dressing becomes saturated with bloody drainage, is it because the patient has changed his body position to one that facilitates drainage? Or has new bleeding started? Consider another example: sudden absence of drainage from a pyelolithotomy wound. Could this be because the wound has healed? Not likely. After pyelolithotomy, the kidney continues to secrete urine, but because of the surgery, this urine will drain through the wound rather than through the ureter. After such surgery, then, sudden absence of drainage can mean one of two things: the wound drainage has become clogged by a stone or clot, or the patient has stopped making urine — an ominous sign. (See page 126 for a summary of characteristic findings in wound drainage.)

Examine the incision itself every time you change the dressing. Have its edges remained approximated? Notice especially skin temperature and sensitivity around the incision. If the skin feels unusually warm, a local infection may

NORMAL SURGICAL WOUND DRAINAGE

PROCEDURE	DAY OF SURGERY	1st DAY POSTOP	2nd, 3rd DAY POSTOP	4th DAY TO DISCHARGE
Abdominal-perineal resection	Profuse; serosanguineous; 2 to 4 hours*	Moderate; serosanguineous; 4 to 6 hours	Moderate; serous; 6 to 8 hours	Minimal; serous; 16 to 24 hours
Appendectomy (simple)	Minimal; serous (brownish)	Minimal; serous	None	None
Appendectomy (with rupture)	Moderate; purulent; brown-green; 4 to 6 hours	Moderate; purulent; 8 to 16 hours	Minimal; serous; 24 hours	Minimal; serous; 24 hours
Cholecystectomy (without T-tube to bile bag)	Moderate to large; sanguineous with bile; 3 to 4 hours	Moderate; bile (brown); 4 to 6 hours	Moderate; brown, serous; 6 to 8 hours	Minimal; serous; 16 hours
Colectomy	Moderate; serosanguineous	Small; serous	Minimal; serous	Minimal; serous
Cystectomy	Moderate; serosanguineous; 3 to 4 hours	Small; serous; 8 hours	Minimal; serous; 24 hours	Minimal; serous; none
Gastrectomy	Moderate; serosanguineous; 6 to 8 hours	Moderate; serosanguineous; 6 to 8 hours	Small; serous; 8 to 16 hours	Minimal; serous; 24 hours
Hysterectomy (abdominal)	Minimal; serous	Minimal; serous	None	None
Inguinal herniorrhaphy	Minimal; serous	Minimal; serous	None	None
Nephrectomy; nephroureterectomy	Moderate; sanguineous; 4 to 6 hours	Moderate; serosanguineous; 6 to 8 hours	Minimal; serous; 8 hours	Minimal; serous; 24 hours
Pyelolithotomy	Profuse; serosanguineous (urine); 1 to 2 hours	Profuse; serous (urine); 2 to 4 hours	Profuse; urine; 4 to 6 hours	Moderate to minimal; urine; 6 to 8 hours
Ovarian cystectomy	Minimal; serous	Minimal; serous	Minimal; serous	None
Small bowel resection	Moderate; serosanguineous; 4 to 6 hours	Moderate; serosanguineous; 6 to 8 hours	Small; serous; 8 to 16 hours	Small; serous; 24 hours
Splenectomy	Moderate; sanguineous; 6 to 8 hours	Moderate; serosanguineous; 6 to 8 hours	Small; serous; 24 hours	Minimal; serous; 24 hours

*Time between dressing changes

be developing (though usually not for several days after surgery). When the incision looks purplish and is hard and tender to touch, think of wound hemorrhage. The skin around the incision should be of normal color and turgor, except for the tiny areas around each skin clip or suture; these areas are usually reddened.

Genitourinary assessment

Begin with inspection of the urine as to color, amount, frequency, presence of sediment, and odor. And palpate for bladder size. Also check the patency of ureteral catheters, Foley catheters, or any used for bladder decompression (continuous bladder irrigation). The urine itself, whether voided naturally or by tube, should be yellow and clear, without foul odor. Of course, if surgery has involved the bladder, kidneys, ureters, rectum, or uterus, expect to see some blood in the urine for 12 to 24 hours after surgery.

Next, evaluate urine output. A well-hydrated patient should have normal urinary function — the ability to void an adequate amount of urine (about 200 ml at first voiding) without the need to void again for several hours (unless I.V. fluids are infusing rapidly). If the patient has drainage tubes, normal function means continuous flow of urine (about 30 ml per hour). However, many surgeons consider low urine output for the first 24 hours (800-1500 ml) to be normal because of: fluid restriction before surgery; loss of body fluids due to hyperventilation; diaphoresis; drainage; and increased secretion of ADH due to stress. They expect "surgical diuresis" (mobilization of sequestered fluid) on the second and third postop day, with balanced intake and output at the end of the fourth.

To palpate bladder size, position the patient flat on his back, with the bed as flat as possible. Ask him to relax his abdominal muscles. (Some patients can relax better if given something else to concentrate on such as wiggling the toes on one foot.) Tell the patient what you are going to do and why. Then palpate, using your cupped hand and a rolling motion. If distended, the bladder will feel like a firm, rounded mass in the center of the lower abdomen. Peristalsis temporarily gets stilled by anesthetics and other medications. Abdominal distention, anorexia, nausea, vomiting, and hiccoughs indicate persistent impairment of peristalsis. Normal bowel sounds, the passing of flatus, and a bowel movement confirm the return of normal peristalsis. Often following abdominal surgery, bowel sounds are absent or hypoactive for 24 to 48 hours. Before deciding if bowel sounds are definitely absent, listen for 2 minutes or longer in the right lower quadrant.

Gastrointestinal assessment

Many patients develop *abdominal distention* after abdominal surgery. It results from accumulation of swallowed gas (ice or fluids taken through a straw increase air intake) or air-swallowing to overcome nausea. It's also partially due to manipulation of the bowel during surgery. Some drugs inhibit the smooth musculature of the GI system. This can lead to ileus if left untreated. "Gas pains" and abdominal distention are distressing and can compromise the patient's respirations. To prevent such distention, many patients need decompression with drainage tubes until peristalsis returns. Nasogastric and Miller-Abbott tubes are used to decompress the stomach and intestines. When such tubes are necessary, check them frequently for the amount and kind of drainage and for patency (see opposite page).

You can best recognize abdominal distention by comparing the patient's abdominal girth to his previous measurements. But inspection and percussion of the abdomen also help. In a patient with gaseous distention, you should be able to hear a tympanitic percussion note.

Nausea may be a side effect of anesthetic medications or may be due to psychologic or other factors. For example, it may be a clue to a blocked decompression tube. Or it may simply result from the replacement of dentures while the gag reflex is hyperactive. Sometimes, vomiting occurs because oral intake began before the return of peristalsis. Remember this, because many patients complain of thirst soon after surgery. Relieve such thirst safely by wetting the lips with ice chips until peristalsis returns. Vomiting that *begins* more than 24 hours after surgery usually points to something other than anesthetic medications. When a postoperative patient is vomiting, report what medications he is receiving, along with the amount, color, odor, and consistency of the vomitus. Persistent vomiting is often a symptom of pyloric or intestinal obstruction, peritonitis, or postop ileus.

Hiccoughs, not uncommon, have various causes. Record

NORMAL TUBE DRAINAGE					
TUBE	SUBSTANCE	AMOUNT DAILY	COLOR	ODOR	CONSISTENCY
Foley	Urine	500 to 2500 ml	Yellow	Ammonia	Watery
Gastrostomy	Gastric contents	Up to 1500 ml	Pale yellow-green	Sour	Watery
Hemovac	Wound drainage	Depends on operative procedure	Varies with procedure	None	Variable
Ileal conduit	Urine	500 to 2500 ml	Yellow	Ammonia	Watery, with some mucus initially
Ileostomy	Small bowel contents	Minimal to 500 ml	Brown	Sour, fecal	Initially serous mucous-like, liquid stool
Miller-Abbott	Intestinal	Up to 3000 ml	Dark green to brown	Fecal	Thick
Nasogastric	Gastric contents	Up to 1500 ml	Pale yellow-green	Sour	Watery
T-Tube	Bile	500 ml	Bright yellow to dark green	Acrid	Thick
Suprapubic	Urine	500 to 2500 ml	Yellow	Ammonia	Watery
Ureteral	Urine	750 ml (30 ml/hr)	Yellow	Ammonia	Watery

their presence in your notes. Report persistent hiccoughs.

Assess *bowel sounds* immediately postanesthesia and routinely thereafter. Be sure to auscultate the abdomen *before* you manipulate the abdomen in any way (because manipulation can alter bowel sounds). During auscultation, listen to all four quadrants of the abdomen to determine the frequency and character of the sound. Normally, you can hear clicks and gurgles at a rate of 5 to 34 sounds per minute. High-pitched tinkling sounds suggest intestinal fluid and air under tension in the bowel. Rushes of high-pitched sounds that coincide and reach a crescendo, indicate obstruction. Bowel sounds are absent in patients with hypokalemia and peritonitis.

COMMON POSTOPERATIVE COMPLICATIONS

COMPLICATION	COMMON CAUSES	OCCURRENCE	SIGNS AND SYMPTOMS
Atelectasis	Mucus plug obstructs bronchial passageway; that portion of lung fails to expand	24 to 48 hours	Fever; increased pulse and respirations; cough; dyspnea; cyanosis; malaise; lung dull to percussion
Hemorrhage	*Early:* slipping of ligature or dislodging of clot *Late:* sloughing of clot or tissue; infection; erosion of vessels by drainage tube	*Early:* within 48 hours *Late:* 6th or 7th day postop	Pallor, rise then fall in blood pressure; increased pulse rate; restlessness; cloudy sensorium; dry mouth; warm dry skin. If external — bright red bleeding (fresh) or dark red blood (drainage) evident
Hypostatic pneumonia	Insufficient lung expansion; fluid accumulation; failure to cough up mucus	24 to 48 hours	Fever; increased pulse and respirations; cough; dyspnea; cyanosis; malaise; lung dull to percussion; expectoration of purulent or blood-tinged sputum
Hypoxia	Anesthetics; preop medications; depressed respirations; mucus blocking airway; pain; poor positioning	Variable	Restlessness; tracheal plug; grunting respiratory efforts; perspiration; bounding pulse; increased BP; cyanosis around lips and nail beds
Shock	Loss of fluids and electrolytes; trauma (both physical and psychological); anesthetics; preop medications	Variable	Pallor; decreased blood pressure; increased and weak pulse; cold moist skin; restlessness progressing to lethargy and/or confusion; decreased urine volume
Thrombophlebitis	Venous stasis; irritation of vessel lining (as caused by I.V. lines)	Variable	Dilated vasculature in extremities; edema; tenderness; increased firmness and tension of legs; calf pain on dorsiflexion; redness; skin warm to touch
Wound evisceration	Malnutrition; defective suturing; strain from coughing; sneezing	Between 6 to 8 days postop	Separation of wound edges with protrusion of organs
Wound dehiscence	Same as above	Same as above	Separation of wound edges *without* protrusion of organs.
Wound infection	Poor sterile technique	3 to 6 days postop	Increasing pain in incision; localized heat; redness; swelling; purulent exudate; fever; chills; headache; anorexia; malaise
Oliguria	Hypovolemia; decreased cardiac output; renal failure due to acute tubular necrosis	Variable	Urine less than 30 ml/hr

Check the patient's stool for color, amount, odor, and consistency. A tan or light-colored stool after a cholecystectomy suggests an absence of bile. Black or red-colored stool (a sign of bleeding) is always significant, particularly after intestinal surgery. Guaiac-test all drainage for accurate assessment of the presence of blood. Remember that stool also drains from colostomies, ileostomies, and sometimes from wounds and other drainage systems.

Monitor intravenous therapy, including arterial and venous lines, closely. Frequently check the I.V. needle or catheter for patency. Also, inspect the site of infusion and surrounding tissue for signs of tissue damage, infiltrations, and phlebitis.

When assessment is complete

Had you completed the preceding assessment by system on Mr. Scott, your notes would read as follows:

Circulatory:	Skin: pink, warm, dry; BP, 114/80; AP, 88 regular.
Respiratory:	Respirations slow, deep, even, effective.
Neurologic:	Muscular coordination intact; recognized wife; groggy conversation.
Wound:	Dressing dry and intact with no through drainage.
GI:	Abdomen flat (no bladder distention). Nasogastric tube patent with clear watery reflux, no nausea. I.V. infusing well.
GU:	Oliguria, flank pain.

The data collected by this efficient and thorough method fell within expected ranges for Mr. Scott. So he will be reassessed at 5- to 10-minute intervals for 1 hour, then every 15 minutes until he remains stable (vital signs and overall assessment within expected ranges for at least 1 hour). Afterward, assessment intervals can be prolonged in a "times four" sequence: Check the patient every 15 minutes x4; every 30 minutes x4; every hour x4; and then every 4 hours. Another helpful rule of thumb is to check any system, varying from normal, every 15 to 30 minutes. If you see no changes in four consecutive checks, and the patient's vital signs are normal, you can consider the patient stable.

Remember that reliable communication of your findings to other staff members is just as important as the assessment itself. Systematic assessment leads smoothly to accurate and complete charting and reporting. When consulting a doctor or another nurse, if you have all the information you gathered in a systematic format, you can easily state the patient's condition concisely and accurately and be prepared to ask and answer questions intelligently.

One difficulty you may have is deciding which symptoms are significant and which are not. To help you decide, remember these rules of thumb:

• Symptoms radically deviant from the norm are always significant.

• Any symptom that recurs consistently or becomes more severe is important.

• The system presenting the most rapidly changing data is likely to have the most serious problem even though its cause may be in another system.

Your goals of caring for the postanesthetic patient are fundamental: Maintain a patent airway. Watch carefully for signs of respiratory obstruction, shock, and hemorrhage (the most common postanesthetic complications). Position the patient carefully for both comfort and safety. Maintain the proper function of drainage apparatus and other equipment. Finally, accurately perform and record a system-by-system assessment.

10

GI BLEEDING and PANCREATITIS
Battling lethal crises

BY EDWINA A. McCONNELL, RN, MS

THE CRITICALLY ILL PATIENT with a gastrointestinal problem is likely to have GI bleeding or acute pancreatitis. In either case your nursing care will be demanding and complex. Do you know what to include in your initial and continued assessment of such patients? What laboratory tests are likely to be ordered? What treatments you may give? This chapter will give you some helpful insights.

Mr. Meyers, a 71-year-old retired welder, came to the emergency department by ambulance after vomiting bright red blood for 2 hours. The day before, he had vomited "coffee-ground" colored material. At admission, he complained of feeling extremely light-headed. He told the nurse he had arthritis for which he regularly took aspirin. His arthritis had been much worse lately, so he'd been taking more aspirin than usual. He had not had bloody or melenic stools. The admitting diagnosis: erosive gastritis.

The E.D. staff inserted a nasogastric tube, which was irrigated with 1500 ml of iced normal saline. The suctioned returns were light to dark red with clots. The staff drew blood for a CBC with platelet count, prothrombin time, partial thromboplastin time, and type and cross match for 4 units of

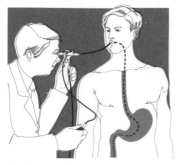

Inside story

In gastroscopy (also called gastric endoscopy), a lighted scope provides a direct view of the gastric mucosa, including lesions too superficial to be seen with X-rays.

The newer, flexible tubes—called fiberscopes—are easier to insert, more comfortable for the patient, and less likely to cause perforations than the older, rigid tubes they replace. Many have cameras that provide still photographs or motion studies of stomach motility.

Prepare a stable patient who is to undergo elective endoscopy by having him fast, and by explaining the procedure in detail so he can cooperate. Just before the test, you may give sedatives, narcotics, or atropine; and, after removing the patient's dentures you may spray procaine on the posterior pharynx to inhibit the gag reflex.

In emergency endoscopy, accompany the patient to X-ray and monitor his vital signs throughout the procedure.

After gastroscopy, watch for signs of perforation (crepitus, fever, or pleural effusion) and for anesthetic reactions. Withhold food and drink until the gag returns (usually 3 to 4 hours after scoping). Relieve hoarseness or sore throat with saline gargles or lozenges.

packed red cells (of which Mr. Meyers received 1 in the E.D.).

At arrival on the medical/surgical unit, his vital signs were: temperature, 98.2° F. (36.8° C.); pulse, 104; respirations, 17; and blood pressure, 148/80. His skin was warm and dry, and he was alert and oriented. An I.V. of 5% dextrose in ½ normal saline was infusing at 125 ml per hour. He had a nasogastric tube in place; it was set up for intermittent low suction and irrigation with a total of 2 liters of iced saline with 8 mg of levarterenol (Levophed) in 200 ml of normal saline. Several institutions prefer to use the Ewald tube. This tube affords better lavage and clot removal, as it contains several large holes at the sides and at the tip. He was also to receive cimetidine (Tagamet) intravenously, 300 mg every 6 hours. He was to have blood drawn for hematocrit determination every 4 hours, a total of six times. The first hematocrit at 1:30 a.m. was 39; 4 hours later, it was down to 35, so he received another unit of packed cells. He also received Maalox, 30 ml every hour, via nasogastric tube. The tube was clamped for 15 minutes after each antacid installation.

The next day, gastroscopy showed active bleeding from a site near a hiatus hernia, but no definite lesion. After his gastroscopy, the nurse kept the patient NPO and watched him closely to prevent aspiration until his gag reflex returned. Later that day, Mr. Meyers was taken to X-ray for celiac angiography with vasopressin (Pitressin) infusion at the rate of 0.5 ml/minute. Near the end of the procedure, he vomited about 1000 ml of red blood and was transferred immediately to the surgical intensive care unit (SICU). Vasopressin was infusing in the proximal celiac artery.

In SICU, he received 2 units of packed cells, 1 unit of whole blood, and 2 units of fresh frozen plasma. His nasogastric tube was lavaged with 16 mg of levarterenol (Levophed) in 400 ml of normal saline. He received oxygen at 3L/minute via nasal prongs. That day, his skin was cool to touch and looked pale (vital signs: temperature, 100.4° F. [38° C.] rectally; pulse, 72; respirations, 24; blood pressure, 150/80). Urine via Foley catheter; 30 to 40 ml/hour. The vasopressin infusion site showed no evidence of bleeding, and his pulses and circulation were adequate.

On the third day after admission, Mr. Meyers' condition stabilized. His blood pressure was 120/70; pulse, 70; hematocrit, 36.5; urinary output was more than adequate. And he had normal bowel sounds. On the fourth day, he continued to improve, so his Foley catheter and nasogastric tube were removed. After another 24 hours, he was transferred to the general surgical floor where he completed his recovery. The day before discharge, Mr. Meyers had an upper GI series, which showed a small peptic ulcer. He was discharged after receiving detailed instructions about diet and medications, and cautioned not to use aspirin.

As you can see from this case, only after all supportive steps have been taken and the patient's condition has stabilized, can the doctor try to find out the cause of the bleeding. Mr. Meyers' confirming upper GI series was done when he had recovered from his bleeding episode and was almost ready for discharge.

What causes GI bleeding?

Roughly 80% of all cases of upper GI bleeding are due to ulcers of the duodenum, esophagus, and stomach; 10% to 20%, to erosive gastritis; and the remaining 5% to esophageal varices. Rarer causes include Mallory-Weiss syndrome (laceration of the mucosa at the junction of the esophagus and stomach as a result of severe vomiting) and gastric cancer.

How does such bleeding happen? In ulcers, erosion of a blood vessel causes the bleeding; the size of the vessel and the elasticity of its walls determine the amount. Erosive gastritis results from ingestion of irritants such as alcohol, aspirin, and steroids, and from anticoagulants, which induce hemorrhage. Esophageal varices are compensatory collateral vessels resulting from portal hypertension. They are inelastic, tortuous, fragile, and distended, and they have a low pressure tolerance. Therefore, they bleed easily. Some minor provocations can make such varices bleed: regurgitation of stomach acid; swallowing large pieces of semi-chewed food; and increased intra-abdominal pressure from sneezing, coughing, lifting heavy objects, or straining at stool.

Three common causes of *lower GI bleeding* are: anal lesions (fissures, fistulas, and hemorrhoids); diseases of the rectum and colon (cancer, ulcerative colitis, and rectal polyps); and diverticuli (most often found in the sigmoid colon).

How does the doctor decide which of these possible causes is actually producing bleeding? He uses clues from the history, a physical examination, and diagnostic tests.

Color's a clue

When blood is vomited or aspirated by nasogastric tube, the stomach or duodenum is almost always the site of bleeding. If the blood is bright red, it's fresh. But if it's dark red or looks like coffee grounds, it's been in contact with gastric acid for perhaps several hours.

Blood in the stool may occur alone or in association with hematemesis. The color of this blood and the stool can help pinpoint the bleeding site:

Bright red blood only: bleeding in rectum and lower sigmoid

Bright red blood mixed with stool: bleeding below mid-transverse colon

Bright red blood on stool surface: bleeding in rectum and lower sigmoid

Maroon blood with diarrhea: bleeding above mid-transverse colon

Melena with diarrhea: bleeding above ligament of Treitz

Melena without diarrhea: bleeding above mid-transverse colon

Blood and stool mixed with pus: bleeding caused by inflammatory disease of the colon

Occult blood: bleeding anywhere in GI or upper respiratory tract

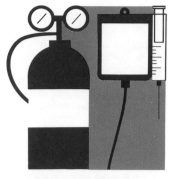

Equipment for nasogastric or Sengstaken-Blakemore tube insertion:
Stethoscope
Sterile irrigation set with bulb syringe
Catheter tip 50-cc syringes for irrigation
10-cc syringe
Emesis basin with ice; large basin
Levine tube; Sengstaken-Blakemore tube
Pressure manometer (mercury aneroid sphygmomanometer)
Gomco (decompression machine)
Water-soluble lubricant
Hemostats, Hoffman clamp, nasal sponge, adaptor, scissors, tape, safety pin
Tincture of benzoin
Disposable towels or drapes
Nonsterile gloves
Bottles of sterile normal saline solution (NSS) for irrigation
Topical anesthetic spray or jelly, such as Lidocaine 4%.

Clues from the history

Never forget to ask the patient what his chief complaint is. Why did he come to the hospital this time? Has he ever had bleeding, peptic ulcer, or chronic liver disease? Has he had a recent nosebleed or a tooth extraction with excessive bleeding? How much alcohol does he drink daily? Does he take aspirin, steroids, or anticoagulants? These drugs are notorious for provoking hemorrhage. Does he have a history of any bleeding disorders? How does he look? Is he jaundiced, pale, or diaphoretic? Does he feel weak or light-headed? Does he vomit blood or pass it by rectum? How much? What color is it? Does he have any abdominal pain? Where? How long? What offers relief?

Since blood that leaks into the GI tract below the duodenum rarely reenters the stomach, vomited blood (hematemesis) nearly always means bleeding somewhere above the ligament of Treitz, at the duodenojejunal junction. As you know, the color of vomited blood varies from bright red to black, depending on the amount of gastric contents at the time of bleeding and on the length of time the blood was in the stomach. Gastric acids oxidize red hemoglobin to brown hematin, changing blood to "coffee grounds" color. So, generally, the shorter the time blood stays in the GI tract, the brighter its color. If the patient's vomited or aspirated blood is bright red, it's fresh; if it's dark red or looks like ground coffee, it's been in contact with gastric acid for perhaps several hours. In either case, the stomach or duodenum is the site of bleeding.

Melena (tarry stools) may appear alone or with hematemesis. However, upper GI hemorrhage that causes hematemesis usually causes melena, too. As little as 60 ml of blood in the gastrointestinal tract produces black, tarry stools. Such melena may persist from 1 to 3 days, depending upon the amount of bleeding; afterward, the stools may remain positive for occult blood an additional 3 to 8 days. Tarry stools are more common with duodenal than gastric ulcers. Passing bright red blood from the rectum usually indicates lower gastrointestinal bleeding. However, in a patient with massive hemorrhage and gastric hypermotility, upper GI bleeding can cause bright red stools. Of course, certain medications and foods also cause black or red stools: iron, charcoal, Pepto-Bismol, and licorice cause black stools; beets cause red or purple stools.

Always ask about epigastric pain relieved by antacids or milk — a pattern that suggests peptic ulcer. A history of alcohol abuse and jaundice suggests chronic liver disease. Specifically ask, too, about any other symptoms — diarrhea, weight loss, abdominal pain, anorexia, heartburn, dysphagia, fever. Any bleeding from other sites such as the skin, mouth, mucous membranes? Any recent problems with nosebleeds or easy bruising? This may point to a primary coagulation disorder.

Physical examination

Inspect the skin and mucous membranes for any signs of bleeding, bruising, pigmentation, and petechiae — any of which might indicate a primary coagulation disorder. Look for signs of liver disease, which would suggest portal hypertension as the cause of bleeding. Does the patient have liver or spleen enlargement, or signs of liver disease? Edema or ascites? Palmar erythema? Spider angiomas? Any sign of collateral abdominal venous circulation? Gynecomastia, or testicular atrophy? Palpate the abdomen for any areas of tenderness or distention. Unless the stool contains visible blood, always do a guaiac test for occult blood. Remember that bleeding from gastric erosion typically produces no other characteristic physical findings.

Look for signs of shock. Systemic signs of gastrointestinal bleeding usually appear with the sudden loss of 20% or more of the total blood volume (roughly 75 ml/Kg of body weight). Remember, tachycardia and rising respiratory rate are signs of a compensatory attempt to oxygenate the tissues despite decreased blood volume. But orthostatic hypotension is more reliable. A drop in blood pressure greater than 10 mm Hg upon sitting upright and/or 10% increase in pulse rate implies at least a 20% volume depletion. With such depletion, the patient may faint and complain of light-headedness, thirst, and nausea. He may appear restless, anxious, diaphoretic, and confused. When volume depletion reaches 40%, the patient generally experiences tachycardia, a thready, peripheral pulse, and cold, clammy skin. He then tends to look pale and may complain of chills.

What diagnostic tests?

Routine laboratory studies in patients with GI bleeding include

What to do first

Your immediate assessment of a GI bleeder should cover these points:

• *Is the patient in shock?* Even if he's not, he'll need an I.V. to provide access to circulation and for rapid fluid replacement to restore blood volume.

• *How much blood has he lost?* Hypovolemic shock doesn't begin until the patient has lost 20% of his fluid volume. Estimate the amount of blood lost by the degree of shock (see page 138).

• *Check pulse and blood pressure*, the most important vital signs in shock, every 15 minutes until the patient's condition stabilizes.

• *Is he still vomiting blood?* He'll need a nasogastric tube passed so that ice lavage can be used to control the bleeding.

• *Is his skin cool and clammy?* To improve tissue perfusion, he'll probably need oxygen.

• *Get a blood type and cross-match*, along with a hemoglobin and hematocrit determination. Be ready to give transfusions as the patient needs them.

Shock of recognition

You can estimate a patient's blood loss quite accurately from the degree of shock he exhibits:
• Severe shock (systolic pressure below 70, pulse rate greater than 130) indicates a life-threatening loss of blood;
• Moderate shock (systolic pressure between 70 and 90, pulse rate between 110 and 130 beats per minute) usually indicates 25% to 40% blood loss;
• Mild shock (systolic pressure greater than 110) usually indicates blood loss less than 25%.

blood workup (CBC, coagulation studies, serial hematocrit and hemoglobin determinations); liver function tests (BSP, LDH, SGOT, bilirubin, serum proteins, transaminases); renal function tests (BUN and creatinine); and arterial blood-gas determinations. Special tests include endoscopy, selective angiography, upper GI series and rectosigmoid examination. (See page 94 for more about liver function tests.)

Many doctors feel that all possible sites of bleeding must be checked out. GI bleeding doesn't always come from the logically most probable site. At least half of the patients with known cirrhosis may bleed from a site other than varices; two-thirds of those with previous gastric surgery may bleed from lesions other than anastomotic ulcers.

Treatment: Combat shock

Whatever the cause of GI bleeding, its overriding danger is shock. Thus, your goals are to maintain adequate circulating blood volume and tissue perfusion, assess and control bleeding, and avoid complications. To do these things, you must continuously monitor the patient's fluid balance, using his vital signs, urine output, and a complete intake and output record as guides. Initially you'll rapidly infuse lactated Ringer's solution or 5% dextrose in water with normal saline via a #18 angiocath until blood pressure returns to normal. Later, when the patient's blood is cross matched and blood units are available, you may begin blood replacement if hypotension, tachycardia, and blood volume show a need for it (see insert). To counteract *severe* shock even before the patient's blood has been typed and cross matched, you can use standing orders to give plasma or type O, Rh negative blood.

Remember the most important thing to do before giving a blood transfusion: *Make sure you have the right blood and the right patient.* Check and double-check, preferably with another nurse, the patient's name, his ABO group, and Rh status, the patient's identification number, and donor number on blood bag and transfusion slip. If you find the smallest discrepancy, don't give the blood. Notify the blood bank immediately.

Once transfusion has begun, closely watch the patient for any untoward reaction. Any such reaction will usually develop within the first 15 minutes. Generally, transfusion reactions include the following symptoms: dyspnea, hives, mild edema, cough, bronchial wheezing, backache, chills, or headache. If you notice any of these signs or symptoms, stop the infusion immediately and notify the doctor. Remember, coagulation factors may be depleted and, therefore, should be checked after infusion of several units of bank blood. Calcium may also be depleted. This is due to citrate in bank blood binding to calcium, so patient may need supplemental calcium.

Monitoring fluid replacement

Check the bleeding patient's vital signs at least every 15 minutes until he's stable. When fluid replacement is adequate, the pulse, respiratory rate, and blood pressure should return to normal. The patient needs more fluid if he becomes apprehensive, complains of thirst, develops a thready pulse, rapid respiratory rate, or low blood pressure, becomes pale, and has cool, clammy skin. He may also need oxygen (usually 3 to 5 L/minute, via nasal prongs). Arterial blood-gas determinations and hemoglobin and hematocrit will help tell you if he's adequately perfusing enough oxygen.

Serial CVP readings help evaluate fluid replacement. To get consistent readings, hold the manometer at the same level for each reading. Mark this level on the patient's chest with a piece of adhesive tape or Magic Marker. Keep in mind the sources of false readings: lung disease, pulmonary embolism, and blocked or misplaced CVP line. A reading lower than 5 cm H_2O suggests that the patient's blood volume is probably less than normal.

When rapidly infusing large fluid volumes, *check respiratory status* frequently to avoid fluid overload. Auscultate the chest and listen for rales, a sign of fluid accumulation in the alveoli. Also *check hourly urinary output and urine specific gravity*. If urine output is 30 ml/hour, blood pressure is probably adequate to prevent cerebral or cardiac damage. (However, only a 12-lead EKG definitely rules out myocardial ischemia; 1% to 2% of people with GI bleeding die from AMI, due to ischemia from inadequate hemoglobin.) The normal range of urine specific gravity (an index of urine concentration) is between 1.003 and 1.030. If the reading is 1.030 or higher, fluid replacement is probably inadequate. Incidentally, when assessing the patient's fluid output, don't forget to include the number, frequency, color, and consistency of his stools, including liquid bowel movements. Also check his bowel sounds.

Blood:
Fresh, stored, or frozen

Fresh blood offers an advantage over stored blood, because it contains more clotting factors and 2, 3 DPG (diphosphoglyceric acid) which facilitates release of oxygen from the hemoglobin molecule, delivering more oxygen to the tissues.

However, stored blood is more readily available, so this is what patients usually receive in transfusion. Actually, most patients who need transfusions should receive not whole stored blood, but packed red blood cells. These lessen the chance of circulatory overload, reduce the risk of serum hepatitis, and of reactions to plasma antigens, and introduce less sodium, potassium, ammonia, and citrate into the bloodstream. Supplement stored blood with fresh frozen plasma and platelets to supply clotting factors. Coagulation studies tell when these are needed.

Another thing to remember about stored blood: Its citrate preservative tends to bind serum calcium, and the resulting hypocalcemia can cause tetany. So, you may need to supplement with calcium gluconate after infusing every 3 or 4 units of stored blood. If the citrate metabolizes to lactic acid, metabolic acidosis is possible.

Use normal saline when infusing blood. Don't mix blood with fluids containing dextrose or calcium. Dextrose causes red cells to clump, swell, and hemolyze; calcium (in lactated Ringer's, for example), may cause the blood to clot.

The Sengstaken-Blakemore tube

This is a triple lumen tube with an esophageal and gastric balloon which controls bleeding esophageal varices by providing direct tamponade. The doctor inserts this tube, positioning the balloons at the bleeding site.

Once the tube is in place, the gastric balloon is inflated with 150 to 200 cc of air via an air-intake port, and the intake port is closed with a screw clamp. Traction is then applied to the tube, by pulling and taping it tightly to a nasal foam pad or football helmet, until the balloon is against the cardia of the stomach.

Proper nursing care is essential:

• Keep suction equipment handy and use it frequently. Often, another tube is inserted into the esophagus and connected to an intermittent suction machine for this purpose.

• Prevent pressure ulcerations and necrosis. Don't tape the tube so tightly that it puts pressure on the patient's face. Give good skin care.

• Monitor electrolytes, and check the complete blood count with differential and arterial blood gases.

• Give oral care frequently. Clean the patient's nostrils often, and lubricate them with water-soluble ointment. Make sure he has a basin and tissues for oral secretions.

• If the patient is restless, you may have to restrain his hands to keep him from removing the tube.

The nasogastric tube

Since a nasogastric tube is used often in GI bleeding, you should know how to insert

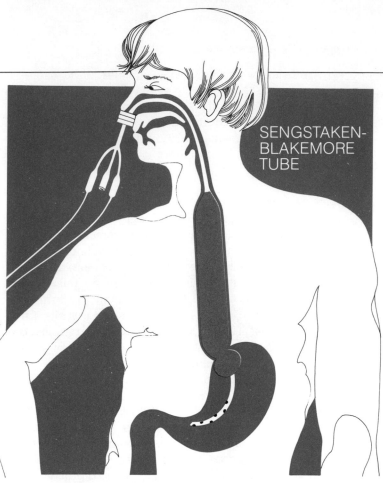

SENGSTAKEN-BLAKEMORE TUBE

one. If you're going to use a red rubber catheter, first chill it in ice for about three minutes to make it less pliable and easier to insert. Most polyethylene tubing is rigid and doesn't need chilling. Watch out—a too-stiff catheter inserted too forcefully can damage the mucous membrane.

Before inserting the tube, lubricate it with a water-soluble agent. Don't use glycerin, which tends to harden rubber tubes. And don't use mineral oil or petroleum, since these can cause acute pulmonary changes or lipid pneumonia.

In patients with a nasal deformity or head injury, insert the tube orally. In other patients, insert it nasally. To do this in semiconscious or comatose patients, raise the head of the bed to a semi- or high-Fowler's position. Tilt the patient's head forward so his chin is in line with his sternal notch. Insert an oral airway, so the patient's tongue doesn't obstruct the pharynx. Advance the tube between respirations. To facilitate insertion, an assistant can stroke downward on the patient's neck.

In conscious patients, elevate

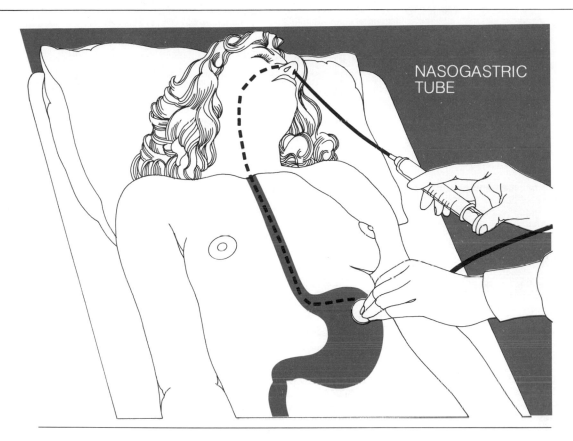

NASOGASTRIC TUBE

the head of the bed 30 to 45 degrees. Tilt the head as with semiconscious patients.

Always insert the tube gently. To prevent gagging, have the conscious patient continually suck on a straw, sip water, or chew ice chips.

After you have inserted the tube, ask the patient to speak. If he can't, the tube is coiled in the larynx. Remove it carefully and reinsert it. Once you have it correctly placed, aspirate with a 50-cc catheter tip or bulb syringe; aspirated gastric contents mean the tube is in the stomach. To double check,

listen with your stethoscope over the patient's abdomen (see above) as you insert 10 to 15 cc of air into the tube. Do you hear a loud whoosh? The tube is in the stomach.

Hold the proximal end of the tube to your ear and listen for airflow. *Never* place this end of the tube into a glass of water, or the patient may aspirate.

Also check for correct tube placement before each feeding and each instillation of antacids. After instilling an antacid, always flush with water afterward to keep the tube patent.

Poor drainage or lack of reflux

suggests that the tube may be coiled in the esophagus, or against the stomach wall. Pulling back on the tube slightly or advancing it may help. If this doesn't work, try repositioning the patient. If there's still no drainage, withdraw the tube completely and reinsert it.

To prevent pressure necrosis or permanently disfiguring sores, don't overtape the tube. To prevent infection, cleanse the patient's mouth frequently. Keep the patient well hydrated, and offer anesthetic throat disks or lozenges to help prevent mucosal irritation.

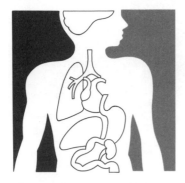

What causes pancreatitis?
The exact causes of acute pancreatitis remain unknown, but it has been linked with several conditions:
● Alcoholism
● Gallbladder or other biliary tract diseases
● Infections originating in the bloodstream, such as scarlet fever or mumps; or in the intestine, such as staphylococcic food poisoning
● Abdominal trauma or surgery
● Hyperlipidemia or hyperparathyroidism
● Use of corticosteroids, thiazide diuretics, azathioprine, or sulfasalazine
● Overindulgence in fatty foods several hours before the attack.

A "churning" sound indicates that a moderate amount of blood is producing a peristaltic bolus.

Nasogastric lavage essential
Any patient who has vomited blood will have a nasogastric tube to empty his stomach, assess bleeding, and give access for gastric lavage and antacid treatment. Keep this tube patent at all times, and record the intake and output accurately; note the color and consistency of the aspirate. Also, know exactly how much irrigant you instill and how much you aspirate to measure and record the amount of bleeding.

For lavage, you can use iced saline or iced saline with Levophed. Iced water should not be used, as it may cause excessive loss of electrolytes from the stomach. Before beginning lavage, make sure the tube is in the stomach. Use 200 ml of iced saline and allow it to remain in the stomach for at least 1 to 2 minutes before suctioning; that encourages vasoconstriction of bleeding vessels and promotes fluid flow through the tube. Manual irrigation clears clots more effectively than does intermittent suction. The usual dosage of levarterenol (Levophed) for lavage: 2 to 4 ampules per 1000 ml of normal saline. Levophed gets absorbed in the stomach and transported via the portal system to the liver, where it's metabolized without producing systemic effects.

You may also use the nasogastric tube to administer antacids, such as Maalox, or a low-sodium antacid such as Amphogel, every 1 to 2 hours. Remember the alkali antacids are nonabsorbable, so don't consider them part of the patient's intake (unlike milk, with which they are sometimes alternated). After instilling an antacid, flush the tube with 30 ml of water to prevent buildup of residue which could block the tube. Be sure to add this water to the patient's daily fluid intake.

Intravenous vasopressin (Pitressin) is used mostly to control bleeding esophageal varices, but can be used to slow arterial bleeding anywhere in the gastrointestinal tract. The dosage: 20 to 50 units of aqueous vasopressin in 100 to 200 ml of 5% dextrose in water infused over 30 to 40 minutes. Or it may be given continuously, 0.2 unit per minute. Vasopressin usually causes diffuse arterial vasoconstriction and decreased portal pressure. Its side effects may include abdominal colic, facial pallor, discomfort, and sudden bowel evacuation. Because of its strong and diffuse arterial vasoconstrictive action, it's contraindicated in patients with a coronary artery disease.

Vasopressin may also be infused intra-arterially to control variceal and other gastrointestinal bleeding. But first, a preliminary arteriogram (via the superior mesenteric or celiac artery) must locate the bleeding site. Then, the vasopressin can be given via an infusion pump at 0.05 to 0.1 units per minute for one to several days. The infusion rate can be increased until bleeding comes under control, but should not exceed 0.4 unit per minute (faster infusion may cause total vascular occlusion). Warn the patient to keep his leg straight during intra-arterial infusion to avoid dislodging the catheter. Monitor this therapy by observing gastric aspirant and taking serial vital signs and hematocrit and hemoglobin determinations. The dose should be tapered over 24 hours as the bleeding slows, and the catheter kept in place for 24 hours postbleeding in case vasopressin needs to be restarted.

After the arterial catheter is removed, the patient should keep his leg immobile for 8 to 12 hours. Check the puncture site for hemorrhage and discoloration, and his upper thigh for increasing size. You may apply a sandbag, icebag, or pressure dressing to prevent bleeding.

Check the popliteal, posterior tibial, and dorsalis pedis pulses and assess the motor and sensory function of the leg, as well as its color and temperature. Compare your findings in the leg used for infusion with those of the other leg. Repeat these checks every 15 minutes for 1 hour; then every 30 minutes for 2 hours; every hour for 4 hours; and finally every 2 hours for 4 hours, and every 4 hours thereafter.

When vasopressin fails
If vasopressin fails to control esophageal bleeding, the doctor may consider an esophageal ballon tamponade using a Sengstaken-Blakemore tube. That can control bleeding by compressing bleeding sites (see pages 140 and 141).

Three severe complications may follow use of the Sengstaken-Blakemore tube; esophageal rupture; tube ascension and regurgitation; and aspiration of gastric contents. Signs of esophageal rupture are rapidly developing back pain, shock, pain in the upper abdomen, and fluid in the chest. If the gastric balloon ruptures, the entire tube may rise into the patient's nasopharynx and completely obstruct his airway. If

When surgery?
Patients suffering from gastrointestinal bleeding are likely to require surgery in the following instances:
• When, though stable, and despite vigorous therapy, they continue to bleed (even a little) for 48 hours.
• When they are debilitated, but continue bleeding for 24 hours.
• When they stop bleeding, but require 3 more units of blood within 24 hours of stabilization.
• When, 3 or 4 days after stabilization, they start bleeding again, massively enough to experience shock.
• When they develop a perforation. This is the most urgent indication for surgery; symptoms include severe pain, board-like abdominal rigidity, and X-ray findings of air under the diaphragm.

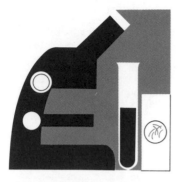

Lab values in pancreatitis
Serum amylase: elevated—
greater than 500 to 2000 Somogyi units/100 ml; rises in 48
to 72 hours and decreases by
the third day of the attack.
(Serum amylase levels may also
be elevated in patients with
mumps or spasm of the sphincter of Oddi; or who have received certain dyes and drugs
including morphine.) So draw
blood sample for this test *before*
all other diagnostic or
therapeutic measures.
Urine amylase: elevated—more
than 2 to 50 Wohlemuth
units/ml (single specimen); or,
(continued)

you see a patient developing acute respiratory distress, deflate the balloon and cut the tube if you have to, but remove the entire tube immediately! To cope with this emergency, keep a pair of scissors handy at the patient's bedside. If esophageal tamponade fails to control GI bleeding, surgery may be indicated.

Pancreatitis: Medical crisis!

Pancreatitis, an acute inflammation of the pancreas, is often associated with alcoholism and biliary tract disease. The fundamental mechanism in pancreatitis appears to be autodigestion of pancreatic tissue and blood vessels by pancreatic enzymes. But no one knows exactly what releases or activates these enzymes. Once released, pancreatic enzymes destroy tissues and blood vessels, causing fat necrosis and liquefaction. The result — edematous or hemorrhagic pancreatitis. Edematous pancreatitis is generally self-limiting and subsides within 2 to 3 days. However, hemorrhagic pancreatitis characteristically produces hyperglycemia, hypocalcemia, persistent ileus, and accumulation of necrotic debris in and around the pancreas. It's a medical crisis, fatal in half the patients.

Recognize pancreatitis by the pattern of pain and by the results of certain laboratory tests. The hallmark of pancreatitis: severe upper abdominal pain, possibly radiating to the back to the region of T10 to L2. Such pain may or may not be accompanied by abdominal tenderness. In early pancreatitis, a patient may have only minimal abdominal tenderness; later, in the full-blown stage, he will have general tenderness, muscle spasm, and rigidity. He may also have nausea and vomiting, restlessness, and anxiety.

Diagnostic studies

The following laboratory studies identify acute pancreatitis: WBC and differential blood count; hemoglobin and hematocrit determinations; amylase; electrolytes; lipase; urine amylase; BUN; creatinine; and X-rays of the abdomen (flat and upright). In pancreatitis, the WBC is usually elevated. Hematocrit may be low; if so, monitor arterial blood gases and Hgb and Hct levels often. Start oxygen. Expect electrolyte abnormalities and watch the potassium level carefully. In pancreatitis, excessive tissue necrosis can cause hyperkalemia and acidosis;

on the other hand, vomiting and gastric suctioning can cause hypokalemia. The serum calcium level is also important. Indeed, diminished calcium level correlates with severity of pancreatitis: serum calcium level below 8 mg/100 ml suggests severe pancreatic necrosis. With normal serum albumin, observe a patient with such severe pancreatitis carefully for tetany. And be ready to give calcium gluconate as needed. Also expect to see elevated blood glucose levels since the pancreas produces the body's insulin.

Serum pancreatic enzymes also help diagnose pancreatitis. For example, a serum amylase level higher than 500 units strongly suggests pancreatitis. Remember, however, that acute cholecystitis and perforated peptic ulcer also raise the serum amylase level. In pancreatitis, elevated serum amylase levels are transient. Serum amylase rises to abnormal levels within 8 hours of onset in 90% of patients, but remains elevated only 48 hours. The serum lipase level rises too, paralleling that of serum amylase. But it stays elevated longer, as does the urinary amylase level. Remember to draw a blood specimen for the serum amylase determination before giving a narcotic analgesic. Opiates stimulate the sphincter of Oddi and produce a falsely high amylase reading. How to distinguish between pancreatitis and hyperamylasemia? An amylase/creatinine clearance ratio may be useful. Generally, a ratio of more than 5.5% indicates acute pancreatitis.

Other abnormal findings in pancreatitis: elevated BUN, and abnormal coagulation studies. Chest films may show an elevated diaphragm, pleural effusion, or basilar pneumonia. Abdominal X-rays may show a loop of gas-distended small intestine in the left upper quadrant. All of these findings suggest pancreatitis, but are not in themselves diagnostic.

Treatment of pancreatitis aims to maintain an adequate circulating blood volume, relieve pain, minimize the pancreas' secretory activity, and prevent or treat complications. You can achieve these aims by...

• *Replacing fluid* to maintain adequate circulating volume.

• *Relieving pain.* You'll generally give meperidine hydrochloride (Demerol) or hydromorphone (Dilaudid). Avoid morphine sulfate (Morphine) and its derivatives because they aggravate spasms at the sphincter of Oddi.

• *Promoting pancreatic rest* by giving nothing by mouth and by placing a *nasogastric tube connected to intermittent low*

Lab values in pancreatitis
(continued)
more than 5000 Somogyi units/24 hours (24-hour specimen)
Serum bilirubin: elevated—more than 0.2 to 1.0 mg/100 ml
BUN: elevated—more than 5 to 25 mg/100 ml
Serum calcium: decreased—less than 8.0 mg/100 ml or less than 4.5 to 5.5 mEq/L
Creatinine: elevated—more than 0.5 to 1.5 mg/100 ml
Serum lipase: elevated—more than 0.1 to 1.5 units/ml
Serum lipids: hyperlipidemia—more than 400 to 800 mg/100 ml
Serum potassium: elevated—more than 3.5 to 5.0 mEq/L in excess pancreatic tissue destruction, or decreased (less than 3.5 to 5.0 mEq/L) in nasogastric drainage or vomiting.
Blood sugar: elevated—more than 90 to 120 mg/100 ml (Folin-Wu)
Serum triglycerides: elevated—more than 25 to 150 mg/100 ml (Folin-Wu)
WBC (leukocytes): elevated—12,000 to 20,000
(Neutrophils): elevated—more than 50% to 75%.

Pseudocyst

Pseudocyst is a cystic structure containing pancreatic juice, necrotic debris and inflammatory cells which forms outside the pancreas and may include parts of the pancreas or neighboring organs and tissues. It usually occurs 3 to 4 weeks after an episode of acute pancreatitis. Characteristically, it produces aching distress rather than acute pain. Because pseudocyst may rupture into the peritoneal or pleural cavity, the mediastinum, or even into the patient's neck, surgical removal is necessary.

suction. The patient with pancreatitis usually has this tube in place about 48 hours, until bowel activity returns. Make sure the tube is patent and that suction is working properly at all times. This is extremely important because acid gastric contents allowed to accumulate and empty into the duodenum stimulate the pancreas to secrete enzymes.

• *Administering anticholinergics* such as propantheline bromide (Pro-Banthine) and antacids reduce pancreatic secretion and relax the sphincter of Oddi. However, some doctors believe that when the pancreas is resting, anticholinergics have little effect on it. Keep in mind that tachycardia, glaucoma, and intestinal ileus contraindicate the use of anticholinergics. Monitor urine output carefully and report retention immediately. You can give a patient with acute pancreatitis antacids hourly, or cimetidine until the attack subsides. If you give them via nasogastric tube, flush the tube afterward with 30 ml water to prevent buildup of antacid residue. Be sure to include this water in the patient's fluid intake record.

• *Giving antibiotics*. Necrotic tissue provides nutrients for bacterial growth, so many doctors routinely order a broad-spectrum antibiotic (one the liver excretes into the biliary tract). Others prefer to wait for signs of infection before ordering antibiotics.

• *Giving insulin* to keep the pancreas at rest. Because the pancreas helps regulate carbohydrate metabolism (via insulin and pancreatic enzymes) watch for hypo- or hyperglycemia in patients with pancreatitis. Avoid hyperglycemia since it stimulates the pancreas to produce *insulin*. The patient may need small doses of regular insulin as indicated by frequent blood glucose tests and fractional urine tests for sugar and acetone.

The symptoms of acute pancreatitis usually subside after 3 or 4 days. Then the patient is allowed small amounts of clear liquids, and, if he tolerates these, his diet is gradually progressed to a low-fat diet. If he's unable to tolerate oral feedings, he may need to be fed via total parenteral nutrition (TPN) If he has biliary tract disease or a pseudocyst (see margin) that needs drainage, the patient with acute pancreatitis may need surgery.

11

THYROID and ADRENAL CRISES
Overcoming endocrine imbalances

BY CATHERINE D. GAROFANO, RN, BS

ENDOCRINE DISORDERS don't usually make a patient critically ill. But when they do, they can rapidly escalate to life-threatening crises. Thyrotoxicosis and Addison's disease are two such disorders that can deteriorate to catastrophic crises. In each case, your correct nursing assessment and intervention can make a critical difference. How? You can help identify thyroid or adrenal instability so that effective treatment can begin promptly; with correctly chosen supportive measures, you can help keep an unstable patient from deteriorating; and finally, the patient-teaching you provide can help a patient maintain stability once his disorder has been controlled.

Mrs. Munoz, 26 years old, was hospitalized because of tachycardia, weight loss, weakness, and unusual irritability. When she arrived, her vital signs were: temperature, 99° F. (37.2° C.); pulse, 128 and regular; respirations, 26; and blood pressure, 150/60. Her skin was smooth; her hair finely textured. Her eyes were sensitive to light and looked unusually prominent. Coagulated blood count (CBC) was within normal limits. Because of her clinical state and prominent eyes, the doctor suspected hyperthyroidism and ordered thyroid function tests. Their results were: ratio of T_3 (triiodothyronine) uptake, 1.6;

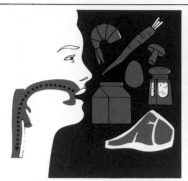

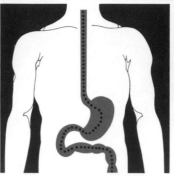

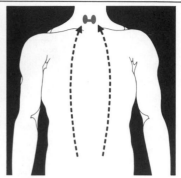

1. Iodine is ingested in sea-foods, vegetables, eggs and dairy products, meat, and io-dized salt.

2. These foods are digested and the iodine they contain is ab-sorbed into the blood from the gut.

3. Iodine travels through the bloodstream and becomes con-centrated within the thyroid gland.

T_4 (thyroxine), 15 mcg/dl; and T_3, 200 mg/dl.

Mrs. Munoz said she'd been feeling fine until 5 months earlier, when her 2-month-old baby died suddenly (sudden infant death syndrome). After this severe emotional shock, she noticed an increase in appetite, but instead of gaining weight she got thinner. She was also cranky much of the time. At first she ignored these symptoms and told herself they were the result of the stress she was under on a new job she'd taken to "keep busy" after her baby's death. But when she also began to experience palpitations, she decided to see a doctor. Mrs. Munoz's symptoms, history, and physical assessment, and the results of her lab tests all pointed to one diagnosis: thyrotoxicosis due to Graves' disease.

What causes thyrotoxicosis?
Thyrotoxicosis or hyperthyroidism results from the overproduction of the thyroid hormones, thyroxine (T_4) and triiodothyronine (T_3). Such overproduction may result from rare thyrotropin-stimulating hormone (TSH)-producing tumors, Graves' disease, nodules, and may even be self-induced, as when healthy persons covertly take thyroid supplements to lose weight. In any case, the cause is over production of thyroid hormone. The patient shows accelerated metabolism with increased oxygen consumption, and heat production, utilization of proteins, carbohydrates, and fats. Such hypermetabolism may vary from mild to extremely severe—the latter, a life-threatening condition called "thyroid storm."

In Mrs. Munoz, thyrotoxicosis stemmed from Graves' disease, an autoimmune disorder often triggered by emotional stress. Graves' disease is the most common cause of thyrotox-icosis. It may occur alone—but is sometimes seen with myasthenia gravis, Addison's, or autoimmune diseases. Its chief symptoms?—nervousness, palpitation, fatigue, weakness, weight loss, heat intolerance and excessive sweating, menstrual changes, tremors, lid re-traction, bulging eyes, and shortened tendon reflex time. The thyroid gland, which is located in the neck, may be visibly enlarged or readily palpable. Graves' disease is more common in women than in men and usually occurs in patients whose family history is positive for

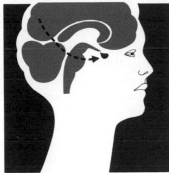

4. Meanwhile, the hypothalamus synthesizes thyrotropin releasing factor (TRF), which travels to the pituitary gland.

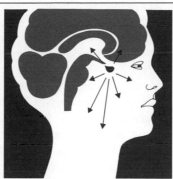

5. Here TRF stimulates the production and release of thyrotropin stimulating hormone (TSH).

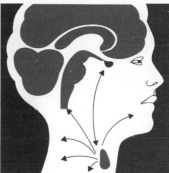

6. TSH then travels to the thyroid gland where it stimulates synthesis of T_4 and T_3 from iodine and their release.

goiter or some other kind of thyroid gland disorder.

How to recognize it?

Watch for characteristic eye changes. These can develop before any clinical or laboratory evidence of thyrotoxic disease. Infiltration of the retro-orbital and periorbital tissues with fluid and polysaccharides produces exophthalmos, the typical "thyroid stare" so often associated with Graves' disease. Another telling clue is pretibial myxedema, edema, and erythema of the subcutaneous tissues over the tibia. Blood pressure may be normal, but usually the systolic is elevated and the diastolic lowered, giving a high pulse pressure.

Mrs. Munoz's thyrotoxicosis was easy to treat because it was recognized so promptly. Her doctor prescribed bedrest to help reduce her metabolic rate; a high-calorie diet (frequent snacks and milkshakes) to overcome her weight loss; and radioactive ablation of the thyroid gland with radioactive iodine. To ease her distressing tachycardia until that treatment could reduce the amount of circulating thyroid hormone (usually about 6 to 12 weeks) her doctor prescribed propranolol. Mrs. Munoz responded to this treatment well and was discharged a week later.

Radioactive ablation of the thyroid gland or antithyroid drugs do usually bring thyroid hormone production under control. But until they do, any extra stimulation or stress, such as an intercurrent illness, could push the unstable thyrotoxic patient into thyroid storm—a perilous condition that's much more difficult to treat. So resist the temptation to underestimate thyrotoxicosis, even if the patient seems to be doing well. Monitor vital signs, stay alert for rising metabolic rate, and protect the patient from overstimulation, stress, and infection.

If you don't, you may find yourself coping unexpectedly with a patient like Mrs. Taylor. A 48-year-old retired teacher, Mrs. Taylor was hospitalized soon after Mrs. Munoz. She too had had clear warnings of severe hyperthyroidism but attributed her symptoms to menopause. Instead of seeking immediate medical help, she'd just kept hoping they'd eventually go away.

Actually, Mrs. Taylor's symptoms were not only easy to see, they were impossible to ignore. Her family reported that she'd been in a state of perpetual motion, constantly cleaning the house or working in her flower garden. She talked incessantly, even when no one was listening. When she did finally sit down, it wasn't long before she popped up again, finding something else to do. She had no problem sleeping most nights but always woke up feeling tired, and she had lost over 20 pounds. Although her family begged her to see a doctor, she refused, and her condition continued to deteriorate for several months. The weekend before she was hospitalized, Mrs. Taylor developed a cold, which rapidly progressed to a severe productive cough, chills, and a fever of 104° F. (40° C.). She also developed diarrhea, and was nauseated and disoriented. Her husband called their family doctor, who arranged for immediate admission to the hospital.

At admission, her vital signs were: temperature, 105.2° F. (40.6° C.); pulse, 160 and regular; respirations, 30; and blood pressure, 110/40. Her face was flushed, and her tissue turgor was poor. We began intravenous glucose infusion immediately. Because her high fever suggested fulminating infection, we took samples for blood, sputum, and urine cultures and began antibiotic therapy. Fortunately, from the history her family provided, her doctor suspected an underlying disorder and arranged an endocrine consultation. The endocrinologist ordered serum thyroid function studies but, after seeing Mrs. Taylor, proceeded to treat her for thyroid storm without waiting for lab results, and correctly so. Unless properly and promptly treated, thyroid storm can lead to coma, vascular collapse, and death. Moreover, although thyroid storm is a life-threatening exaggeration of all the signs and symptoms of thyrotoxicosis, it does not produce serum T_4 and T_3 elevations any higher than those in uncomplicated hyperthyroidism. So thyroid storm is diagnosed on a purely clinical level, with careful reference to recent history.

Weathering thyroid storm

Had Mrs. Taylor sought medical attention earlier, diagnosis and treatment could have prevented this serious, but rare, complication of thyrotoxicosis. But she was now in full-blown thyroid storm and needed aggressive therapy with beta adrenergic blockers (propranolol and cardiac glycosides such as digoxin), sedatives and narcotics to reduce her metabolic rate, and antithyroid drugs (methimazole [Tapazole] and propylthiouracil) to reduce thyroid hormone production. Unfortunately, for the critically ill patient, antithyroid drugs can't be given parenterally but are given as soon as oral intake is possible. Mrs. Taylor improved enough to receive treatment with Tapazole on the third day after admission. And, as such patients usually do, she began to show marked improvement in hypermetabolic symptoms within hours after therapy began. Many patients in thyroid storm also need to receive steroids to combat the overwhelming stress extreme hypermetabolism causes. Mrs. Taylor received hydrocortisone, 300 mg I.V., over 24 hours. As her condition stabilized, this was gradually tapered over 4 days.

Supportive measures

In a patient with hyperthermia, such as Mrs. Taylor, alcohol sponges, ice packs, and cooling blankets (when available) can help bring down body temperature. Maintain the airway, by an endotracheal tube when necessary, and give oxygen as needed. Generally, the severely thyrotoxic patient needs intravenous glucose and vitamins and, if severely wasted, may need total parenteral nutrition. To prevent corneal ulceration in patients with proptosis, keep the eyes moist at all times. Use artificial tears every 4 to 6 hours p.r.n., or place saline-soaked eye pads over the eyes.

Monitor vital signs frequently. Increased thyroid hormone production greatly affects the cardiovascular system, so watch for increased cardiac rate and rhythm, increased urinary output, and elevated arterial blood pressure. A high pulse rate is common and may go as high as 160. Untreated, these cardiovascular changes can progress to atrial arrhythmias, and eventual cardiac output failure, accompanied by hypotension and dyspnea.

Also, check the patient's temperature frequently. Heat intolerance accompanied by profuse sweating is common, but you can help prevent dehydration by promoting adequate ventilation, rest, and fluid intake.

Expect irritability

Thyrotoxic patients are usually irritable and anxious. In fact, the personality and physical changes they experience may lead

Drugs used in thyrotoxicosis

BETA ADRENERGIC BLOCKERS: control signs and symptoms of hyperthyroidism resulting from increased sympathetic activity, such as tachycardia and thyroid stare:
propranolol (Inderal)
Dose—(initially) P.O.: 20 mg q.i.d., may gradually increase every third day until therapeutic level reached. In crisis: 1 mg I.V. q4h; or P.O. 40 mg q6h.

ANTITHYROID DRUGS: inhibit synthesis of thyroid hormones
methimazole (Tapazole)
Dose—P.O.: 5 mg t.i.d. in mild cases, 10 to 15 mg t.i.d. in moderately severe cases, and 20 mg t.i.d. in severe cases. Maximum 150 mg daily. Maintain at 5 mg daily, b.i.d., or t.i.d.
propylthiouracil also called PTU (Propyl-Thyracil, Propacil)
Dose—P.O.: adults—100 mg t.i.d., or up to 300 mg q8h in severe cases. Maximum 1500 mg daily. Maintain at 50 mg daily, b.i.d., or t.i.d.; children 6 to 10 years —50 to 100 mg t.i.d.; children over 10 years— 100 mg t.i.d. Maintain at 25 mg t.i.d. to 100 mg b.i.d.

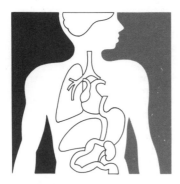

**What causes
adrenal insufficiency?**
In primary adrenal insufficiency
or Addison's disease, the
major adrenal hormones—cortisol, aldosterone, and the
adrenal sex hormones are
inadequate or absent because
of...
• Idiopathic disease (probably
autoimmune)
• Tuberculosis
• Infiltrative or fungal lesions
• Hemorrhage into the adrenal
cortex while taking
anticoagulants.
• Adrenalectomy
• An adrenal toxin such as
ortho-para DDD.
In secondary adrenal insufficiency, inadequate levels
of ACTH produce decreased
cortisol and androgen levels, but
little or no change in
aldosterone secretion; and are
frequently associated with
other pituitary hormone deficiencies. The causes of ACTH
deficiency:
• Pituitary tumors (especially
chromophobe adenomas)
• Postpartum necrosis of the
pituitary gland
• Hypophysectomy
• High dose radiation therapy
to the pituitary gland
• Prolonged or high dose glucocorticoid therapy
• Hypothalamic disease which
causes corticotropin releasing
factor deficiency.

them to believe they have a terminal disease. So don't be
surprised if a thyrotoxic patient complains, "Why bother taking my temperature and pulse so often? I'm going to die anyway!" Do your best to reassure the patient and his family.
Encourage the jittery, restless patient to curtail all nonessential
activity and to stay in bed as much as possible until his condition stabilizes. Before the antithyroid drugs became available, complete bedrest was the only way to manage
thyrotoxicosis. It's still an important adjunct to therapy in
lowering the metabolic rate.

We also gave Mrs. Taylor frequent high-calorie snacks to
help her get a head start on regaining the weight she'd lost.
As the antithyroid drugs began to take hold, she became less
anxious and less irritable, and her family was especially pleased
to see her "seem like herself again." Since she'd been admitted
in a critical condition, her doctor decided to delay definitive
treatment (surgery or ablation of her thyroid gland) until later,
when she regained some of her strength. After 4 weeks of
hospitalization, Mrs. Taylor was discharged and was given
careful instructions for continuing the antithyroid drugs.

Addisonian crisis

"I don't understand it," said Mr. Mueller, whose severely
dehydrated middle-aged wife was admitted to the hospital
with acute abdominal pain, diarrhea, and a fever of 104° F.
(40° C.). He reported that "she had the flu for a few days, but
this morning she suddenly got much worse." The admitting
doctor remembered Mrs. Mueller from a previous hospitalization and immediately suspected acute adrenal insufficiency
(Addisonian crisis). He ordered an immediate intravenous infusion of adrenocortical hormones in normal saline solution.

Mrs. Mueller, it turns out, had been hospitalized about a
year earlier, complaining of chronic weight loss, weakness,
anorexia, light-headedness, and a craving for anything salty.
In fact, her husband said she'd even drink the juice from pickle
jars to satisfy her craving for salt. Her chart showed she'd
been somewhat overweight at that time, with blood pressure
95/50 pulse 86 and regular, and respirations 18. During her
previous hospitalization, her laboratory studies showed low
serum sodium and elevated serum potassium levels. Her CBC
showed slightly increased eosinophils; BUN was 26; and her
chest X-ray was normal. The only obvious sign of primary

adrenal insufficiency was increased pigmentation noticeable around a hysterectomy scar and on her knuckles.

During her previous hospitalization, her 17-hydroxycorticoid and 17-ketosteroid response to ACTH-stimulation was less than 5 mg/24 hours after a 24-hour infusion; and 4 mg/24 hours after 48 hours of continuous infusion. (The normal response: at least 20 mg/24 hours on the first day; at least 40 mg/24 hours on the second day.) Once diagnosed, her Addison's disease was treated with adrenal hormone replacement. Mrs. Mueller made rapid progress and was discharged within a week, with careful instructions about dealing with her disease. But because her disorder seemed so easily controlled, Mrs. Mueller brushed it off as insignificant. She neglected her medication, allowing adrenal insufficiency to deepen into catastrophic illness. We're seeing more cases of adrenal insufficiency like Mrs. Mueller these days, partially because of better diagnostic techniques but also because of increased use of drugs which may be toxic to the adrenals, and of high-dose steroids which suppress normal adrenal tissue and cause it to atrophy.

Expect varying symptoms

Adrenal insufficiency varies quite a lot, with severity of symptoms increasing with the degree of insufficiency. Patients with adrenal insufficiency may develop symptoms of hypoglycemia: sweating, hunger, blurred vision, tremors, restlessness, pallor, muscle twitching, and convulsions. They also develop tachycardia, weakness, or headaches which may result from low blood sugar or low sodium concentration. Such sodium loss causes them to develop irritability, confusion, anxiety, abdominal cramps, tachypnea, and hypotension. Mrs. Mueller's craving for salt was quite typical of adrenal insufficiency and reflected sodium depletion. Other symptoms of adrenal insufficiency include weight loss, anorexia, and fatigue. As adrenal insufficiency becomes more severe, patients develop nausea, vomiting, and diarrhea; some may also lose pubic and axillary hair.

The most obvious sign of primary adrenal insufficiency is hyperpigmentation, especially over the elbows and knuckles, and around scars. It causes patients to appear deeply suntanned, even on parts of the body normally covered with clothes. They may also develop numerous black freckles or

Getting any feedback?
Feedback mechanisms play a big role in maintaining homeostasis. The adrenal-hypothalamic-pituitary feedback mechanism, which controls adrenal cortical secretion, shows how negative feedback comes into play on demand to restore equilibrium.

The hypothalamus releases corticotropin releasing factor (CRF) in response to stress, the sleep-wake cycle, and plasma cortisol levels. This, in turn, stimulates the release of adrenocorticotrophic hormone (ACTH) from the anterior pituitary gland, where it's stored. However, plasma cortisol levels regulate CRF and ACTH release: If cortisol levels are high, CRF (and consequently ACTH) release decreases; if cortisol levels are low, it increases.

What adrenal hormones do

The inner, or medullary, layer of the adrenal gland secretes the catecholamines, epinephrine and norepinephrine; and the outer layer, or cortex, secretes steroid hormones. Steroid hormones include the glucocorticoids, and cortisol; the mineralocorticoid, aldosterone; and androgens, the sex hormones.

Cortisol:
• Influences protein, fat, and carbohydrate metabolism
• Increases the concentration of circulating amino acids
• Promotes the release of fatty acids from adipose tissue and their utilization,
• Stimulates gluconeogenesis and promotes increased concentration of blood glucose.

Aldosterone:
• Stimulates sodium (Na^+) conservation and potassium (K^+) excretion in the renal tubules.
• Promotes water conservation by decreasing urinary output.
• Is released in increased quantities in hyponatremic, hyperkalemic and hypovolemic states.

Adrenal androgens:
• Influence sexual function and the development of axillary and pubic hair in the female.
• Possibly supplement the supply of sex hormones from the gonads in the male.

a bluish-black discoloration of the mucous membranes. Obviously, these pigmentation changes are less noticeable in Blacks and other persons with dark complexions; in such patients, look for these typical changes on the palms, soles of the feet, or mucous membranes and scar tissue.

Patients with adrenal insufficiency usually undergo many diagnostic tests, including 24-hour ACTH (Cortrosyn) stimulation tests. Do your best to schedule these tests to allow the patient adequate rest periods in between. And above all, take time with these patients. Your ability to provide a calm environment, your willingness to answer their questions and to explain the procedures they must undergo can lessen their anxiety, speed their recovery, and help them cope with this permanent disorder.

Drugs for life

Treatment for adrenal insufficiency includes *permanent* replacement therapy with corticosteroids. Cortisone and hydrocortisone, both glucocorticoids, are the most commonly used; however, their mineralocorticoid effect may be inadequate to maintain electrolyte balance, so the mineralocorticoid fludrocortisone (Florinef) may also be needed.

The patient with adrenal insufficiency will need to take these drugs for the rest of his life. How well you educate him about them and his need for them can help ensure the compliance that will keep this disease under control. You can encourage acceptance, for example, by advising taking steroids with meals or snacks to reduce gastric irritation. Also suggest taking steroids in divided doses in the morning and late afternoon to mimic the normal diurnal adrenal rhythm. Warn the patient that steroid dosages vary greatly from one person to another so dosage (especially of the mineralocorticoids) may have to be adjusted several times to find the most suitable dose. Warn the patient not to restrict salt intake without the doctor's consent.

When drug therapy begins, closely monitor sodium and potassium, serum BUN, BS, and CBC levels. Teach the patient to weigh himself frequently and to report any sudden weight loss or gain, since either might signal a need for dosage adjustment. Be sure to tell every patient with adrenal insufficiency to carry a medical identification card or wear a medical alert bracelet, especially during times of dosage adjustment, and to keep handy a kit containing intramuscular cortisone, syringes, and alcohol wipes. Because the patient may need to inject himself with cortisone if nausea or vomiting prevents him from taking it orally, or if severe diarrhea interferes with absorption of oral cortisone, make sure the patient understands exactly when and how to give himself cortisone injections.

Also, tell the patient he'll need to increase his steroid dose, according to the doctor's instruction, during infection, illness, times of stress, and after physical trauma or surgery, including tooth extractions. For instance, a patient with a cold, cough, and a fever of 101° F. (38.3° C.) usually should double his cortisone dose. If the fever reaches 102° F. (39° C.) and persists for more than 24 hours, he should call his doctor for further instructions. Because of this inability to deal with added stress, the patient with adrenal insufficiency needs to be especially careful about avoiding infections and should promptly notify the doctor if he develops an infection. This was where Mrs. Mueller went wrong. While her body was coping with an infection that stretched the limited adrenal steroids available, her diarrhea inhibited intestinal absorption of cortisone. The result: acute adrenal insufficiency. Mrs. Mueller probably could have avoided this acute illness if she had increased her cortisone dose; given herself a cortisone injection to tide her over her bout with the flu; or if she had just called her doctor earlier.

Some women with adrenal insufficiency experience muscle weakness and decreased libido, probably because they lack adrenal androgens. If so, they may benefit from an intramuscular injection of 25 to 50 mg of testosterone every 4 or 5 weeks. Of course, if this causes facial hair growth or other symptoms of masculinization, the dose may need to be lowered or the interval between doses increased.

Patients who follow these suggestions for effective use of steroids will probably maintain good control of Addison's disease. If not, like Mrs. Mueller, they could suddenly find themselves in Addisonian crisis, a critical illness. What then? Untreated, Addisonian crisis leads to vasomotor collapse, hypovolemic shock, coma, and death. So, the immediate plan

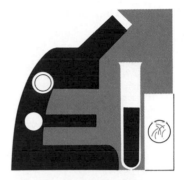

Save that urine!
The ACTH stimulation test can detect deficiencies in adrenal steroid production and reserve. The test measures urinary levels of 17-hydroxycorticoids and 17-ketosteroids after a continuous 24-hour infusion of 50 units of Cortrosyn in saline for 1 or 2 days, or an 8-hour infusion for 4 or 5 days. The patient's urine is collected simultaneously.

In adrenally insufficient patients, these levels are low or absent.(See lab values in adrenal insufficiency, p. 156.)

Since this test is done on the floor, make sure you save the patient's urine. Always keep the urine specimens refrigerated. If no preservatives are added, add 25 ml of glacial acetic acid per 4 qt. container. Make sure the patient isn't taking tetracyclines, multivitamins, or other drugs which may alter test results. Warn the patient, his family, and all shifts not to throw out the urine, or the test will have to be done over.

Lab values in primary adrenal insufficiency
Plasma:
- ACTH: elevated—150 mg/ml
- 17-Ketosteroids: decreased—10 mg/24 hours
- Aldosterone: decreased—0.015 mcg/100 ml
- Sodium (Na): decreased—136 to 145 mEq/L
- Potassium (K): elevated—3.5 to 5.0 mEq/L
- Chloride (Cl): decreased—95 to 109 mEq/L
- Bicarbonate (HCO_3^-): decreased—22 to 26 mEq/L
- Sugar (BS): occasionally decreased—60 to 120 mg/100 ml
- Eosinophil count: increased
- Cortisol: normal or decreased (normal is 5 to 25 mcg/100 ml between 8 and 10 a.m., and 2 to 18 mcg/100 ml between 4 and 6 p.m.)
24-hour urine:
- 17-hydroxycorticosteroids: may be decreased—3.0 to 14.5 mg/24 hours in males; 3.0 to 12.9 mg/24 hours in females
- Aldosterone: decreases—2 to 26 mcg/24 hours.

of action in this crisis is to restore electrolyte balance and fluid volume, and replace steroids.

Mrs. Mueller received an immediate intravenous infusion of normal saline with steroids. She did not receive blood or plasma expanders, although they are often needed in severe hypotension or shock. She received penicillin to counteract the infection. As soon as she was able to take medications orally, she received cortisone acetate 200 to 300 mg P.O./24 hours. When acute adrenal insufficiency produces vasomotor collapse, pressor agents such as norepinephrine (Levophed) and dopamine (Intropin) may also be given, but fortunately Mrs. Mueller didn't need these. Throughout, we also kept a close watch on her vital signs and lab reports. As her condition stabilized, we gradually reduced cortisone acetate dosage to her normal maintenance level.

Preventive teaching
One of the most important things we did for Mrs. Mueller was to educate her and her husband about her illness. We stressed that she couldn't afford to take even minor illnesses lightly, and that she should call her doctor about little things she'd been used to ignoring, such as a persistent cold. We hoped this advice would help Mrs. Mueller keep her illness under control and would stave off another Addisonian crisis.

12

HHNK
Correcting disordered glucose metabolism

BY KAREN E. WITT, RN, BSN, MSN

DO YOU KNOW how to recognize and cope with HHNK—
hyperglycemic hyperosmolar nonketotic coma? If you don't,
you should. It's a life-threatening metabolic derangement, one
you may need to recognize to save the lives of certain patients.
It can occur as a complication in borderline and in unrecog-
nized diabetes, as well as in a variety of medical and surgical
conditions that involve high blood sugar and dehydration. It
has a mortality rate of 60% to 70%!

Consider the unusual case of Mr. Stevens, aged 67, who
came to our hospital with pancreatic carcinoma. Some months
before, he had been found to have elevated blood sugar. Diet
had controlled it until about 3 weeks ago, when he was brought
to the hospital with symptoms characteristic of pancreatic
disease, including colicky pain in the upper right abdomen,
jaundice, and an aversion to food.

Extensive diagnostic studies indicated a pancreatic tumor
obstructing the ductal system. Surgeons did a Whipple procedure that left an unresectable tumor around Mr. Stevens'
portal vein. He did fairly well after this operation, until late
evening of the fourth postop day. He then developed aspiration
pneumonia with a fever of 101° F. (43.8° C.), which required

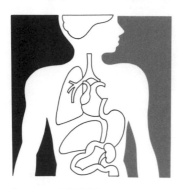

Causes of HHNK
ACUTE ILLNESS: pneumonia;
cerebral vascular accident; infection; pancreatitis; severe
burns.

PRECIPITATING PROCEDURES:
hyperalimentation therapy; peritoneal dialysis; hemodialysis.

DRUGS: (especially those known
to provide insulin insufficiency)
corticosteroids; diuretics (thia-
zides, furosemide); diphenylhydantoin; immunosuppressives.

kanamycin (Kantrex), cephalothin (Keflin), hydrocortisone (Solu-Cortef), and supportive respiratory therapy.

By the fifth day, his blood gases showed a pH 7.58 (normal 7.35 to 7.45), PaCO$_2$ 24.5 (normal 34 to 46 mmHg), PaO$_2$ 41 mmHg (quite below the normal 80 to 105 mmHg). Oxygen therapy was started.

Right after the operation, he had received 5% dextrose in 0.45% saline with potassium chloride (after urinary flow had returned) to keep fluid and electrolyte balance normal. Also, he had received 10 units of regular insulin daily for 2 days; that was changed to 15 units of NPH insulin daily.

Despite the insulin, and although he did not complain of thirst, Mr. Stevens was confused, disoriented, and apprehensive. The nurse discovered him hyperventilating, with respirations 36 a minute. He was lethargic and looked dehydrated. His blood pressure was only 96/50 mmHg; his heart rate, 130 a minute. He seemed to be in classic diabetic ketoacidosis. But his serum acetone was still zero. We notified the doctor.

Lab studies at this point indicated a serum glucose of 720 mg per 100 ml (grossly above the normal 60 to 120 mg) and serum osmolality of 378 mosmol/Kg H$_2$O (above a norm of 280 to 294). With blood glucose and serum solutes this high but without acetone, with a pH not acid but indeed a little alkaline, what kind of ketoacidosis was this? None at all, as you've surmised. The diagnosis was hyperglycemic hyperosmolar nonketotic coma.

A crisis condition

The first concern in HHNK is to restore fluid volume and reduce blood glucose. Mr. Stevens received 50 units of regular insulin (25 units intravenously and 25 subcutaneously), followed by 25 units every 2 hours until his blood sugar level began to come down. Then he received less frequent doses as he needed them.

Under more ordinary circumstances, fluid replacement would have been given at a rate no faster than 30 to 40 ml/Kg to avoid water intoxication—no more than 3200 ml a day for a man whose preoperative weight was 80 Kg (176 lb). But the extreme hyperosmolality and dehydration in HHNK call for extreme measures. So, Mr. Stevens got a full 10.6 liters in 2 days.

Subcutaneous regular insulin was being continued according to Mr. Stevens' blood sugar levels. (Insulin added to I.V.

solutions can be partially inactivated and, in any case, is supplied far too slowly—unless the patient is in shock, when subcutaneous injection becomes useless because of poor tissue perfusion.) The fructose, which can be phosphorylated in the tissues with no need for insulin, was given for cell energy without adding to the hyperglycemic load.

On the eighth postop day, Mr. Stevens' plasma proteins dropped markedly (from 5.1 mg per 100 ml to 1.7), so we began giving intravenous albumin. His blood proteins began to climb back toward normal.

Mr. Stevens also had a low hematocrit, unusual in patients with HHNK. He received 2 units of whole blood to replace blood loss from his operation. After the ninth postop day, his blood glucose generally came down a little (460 mg/100 ml) too. Mr. Stevens even appeared to be recovering from his hyperosmolar coma. He was more alert and no longer dehydrated.

What causes HHNK?

The medical and surgical conditions that precipitate HHNK include those that bring on its forerunner, hyperglycemia: diabetes mellitus, pancreatic disease, pancreatectomy, extensive burns, and glucocorticoid therapy, as well as a variety of acute stress conditions. Like corticoid therapy, stress leads to hyperglycemia through an overproduction of steroids.

Hyperalimentation therapy has sometimes been a factor in HHNK, and so have hemodialysis and peritoneal dialysis, especially when the dialyzing fluid has a high glucose content or remains too long. HHNK occurs most often in adults, but occasionally it happens in children, usually from diabetes, sometimes from heat stroke.

The onset of HHNK is typically insidious, as it was for Mr. Stevens. But once developed, it moves rapidly to a crisis. Early signs in an alert patient usually include polyuria, increased thirst, and a growing impairment of consciousness. Of course, as you are probably thinking, these signs are commonly observed in seriously ill patients of all sorts. And very often you don't have even these signs to go by because the patients are obtunded or perhaps comatose. But this is why it's medically important to follow susceptible patients closely with frequent determinations of blood glucose and electrolytes.

Failure to recognize the risk of HHNK or the syndrome

How HHNK happens

Because glucose is a large molecule, it exerts great osmotic pressure and can attract large shifts of water. In the pronounced hyperglycemia of HHNK, osmosis pulls out intracellular fluid to help equalize the growing osmotic pressure of blood hypertonic with sugar. Intracellular water shifts into the bloodstream, leaving dehydrated cells. At the same time, the sugar overload promotes osmotic diuresis. Without enough water from the outside, the blood becomes even more concentrated and its volume further depleted. The ensuing hypovolemia decreases renal blood flow. This oliguria conserves urine, preserving the remaining extracellular fluid volume to reduce water loss, but it also severely hampers the kidney's excretion of glucose. Without treatment by insulin and fluids, dehydration and hypovolemia become self-perpetuating.

To complicate matters, several of the conditions preceding HHNK are often treated with glucocorticoids. But glucocorticoids may themselves provoke hyperglycemia by gluconeogenesis and by depressing carbohydrate oxidation; they thereby promote diuresis and dehydration. In fact, steroid-induced diabetes persists for some time after steroids are withdrawn. Glucocorticoids may also inhibit the release of antidiuretic hormone. Possibly, they also promote diuresis by reducing tubular capacity to reabsorb water and solutes.

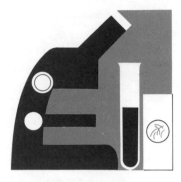

Mr. Stevens' Lab Values

NORMAL
Hematocrit ml/100 ml 40-54
Glucose mg/100 ml 60-120
Serum acetone 0
Urine acetone 0
BUN mg/100 ml 10-20
Sodium mEq/L 136-145
Potassium mEq/L 3.5-5.0
Chloride mEq/L 95-109
Total bilirubin mg/100 ml 0.2-0.9
Serum osmolality
   mosmol/Kg H_2O 280-294
Urine osmolality
   mosmol/Kg H_2O 50-1200
Total protein GM/100 ml 6.6-8.2
PaO_2 mmHg 80-105
$PaCO_2$ 34-45
pH 7.35-7.45
HCO_3—mEq/L 22-26

DPO 5
Hematocrit ml/100 ml 36
Glucose mg/100 ml 370
Serum acetone 0
Urine acetone 0
Sodium mEq/L 145
Potassium mEq/L 4.3
Chloride mEq/L 112
Total bilirubin mg/100 ml 19.8
PaO_2 mmHg 41
$PaCO_2$ 24.5
pH 7.58
HCO_3—mEq/L 22.2

(continued)

itself is bound to contribute to its high mortality rate. It does help to remember the one thing that sets this disorder apart from diabetic ketoacidosis (DKA) and other hyperglycemia-related conditions—minimal or absent ketoacidosis. We can understand HHNK better if we look closely at its separate features.

Hyperglycemia dramatic

In HHNK, hyperglycemia is extreme, linked with the hyper-osmolality responsible for coma. Fasting blood sugars may range from 600 mg per 100 ml to as high as 3000 mg per 100 ml. This high range reflects some breakdown in glucose metabolism, or more glucose intake than the body can metabolize. Clearly, faulty glucose metabolism is the cause in diabetes mellitus and in certain cases of pancreatic dysfunction. In patients with acute pancreatic disease the curtailed supply of endogenous insulin helps elevate the glucose level. In those with known diabetes and in those who have undergone a pancreatectomy, receiving too little insulin can be the cause.

In patients with severe infection or some other acute stress, or those receiving glucocorticoids, you'll find the blood sugar rising through gluconeogenesis. This synthesis of glucose from protein or fat is a natural effect of the adrenal cortex hormones. Steroids also increase the body's resistance to the action of insulin. With this double-barreled effect in mind, you must be extremely vigilant when glucocorticoids are used with a patient such as Mr. Stevens or with any patient who may be predisposed to HHNK.

In burned patients, in hemodialysis, in peritoneal dialysis (when high sugar concentrations are used as the dialyzing fluid and remain long enough for the large sugar molecules to be absorbed), and in hyperalimentation, patients may receive more glucose than they can metabolize. In hyperalimentation the prolonged infusion of high glucose concentrations can lead to pancreatic fatigue because of the sharp, continuous demand on the beta cells to produce insulin. If there is too little insulin for all the glucose to be used in the tissues, it accumulates in the blood. When such buildup is sufficiently prolonged, hyperglycemia will lead to actual degenerative changes in the beta cells. Meanwhile, the HHNK syndrome can develop very quickly if the patient is given too little supplemental water to permit excretion of the glucose by the

CHOOSE YOUR FIRST SKILLBOOK
and save $1.00 on each book you buy when you join the NURSING SKILLBOOK™ series

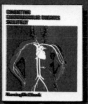

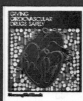
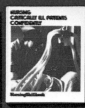
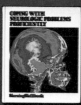
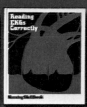
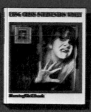

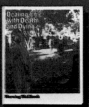
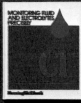

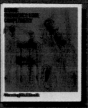
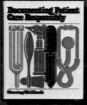

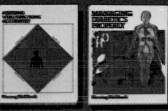

This highly regarded reference series deals thoroughly and professionally with the subjects today's nurse wants—and needs—to know more about! These timely nursing guides draw on the resources and expertise of nursing specialists from throughout the United States to give you complete, detailed answers to all your questions about reading EKGs…crisis intervention…documentation…neurologic disease or injury…and much, much more. And because only you know which of these valuable books will benefit you most, you can select your own introductory volume. Each book contains creative, workable solutions to the problems you face every working day, and the exclusive SKILLCHECK feature lets you test your reactions to tough nursing situations. Each SKILLBOOK offers you: ● 192 fact- and illustration-filled pages ● Convenient 7½" x 9" size ● Durable hardcover binding ● 68,000 words of authoritative, in-depth text ● Complete indexing, so the information you need is always at your fingertips. To discover how membership in the SKILLBOOK series can make you a better nurse, complete and return the attached order card today.

Please send me _____

for a 10-day free examination. If I decide to keep this introductory volume, I agree to pay $8.95 (plus shipping and handling). I understand that I will receive another SKILLBOOK every 2-3 months. Each book costs $8.95 (plus shipping and handling) and comes on a 10-day free-examination basis. There is no minimum number of books I must buy, and I may cancel my subscription at any time, simply by notifying you.

Name _____

Address _____

City _____   State or Province _____   Zip or Mail Code _____

Pa. residents please add 6% sales tax. Offer valid in U.S. and Canada only.   SBBS–1

PROFESSIONAL DATA
Please check one box in each category

1. Personal:
- a ☐ RN
- b ☐ LPN/LVN
- c ☐ Student Nurse
- d ☐ Librarian
- e ☐ Technician
- z ☐ Other _____
  specify

2. Place of Employment:
- a ☐ Hospital
- b ☐ Nursing Home/ECF
- c ☐ Comm. Health Agency
- d ☐ Nursing School
- e ☐ Office
- f ☐ School
- g ☐ Occupational Health
- h ☐ Private Duty
- j ☐ Inactive
- k ☐ Other _____
  specify

3. Position:
- a ☐ Director Nursing Service/Asst.

- b ☐ Administrator or Asst.
- c ☐ Supervisor or Asst
- d ☐ Head Nurse or Asst.
- e ☐ Staff Nurse
- f ☐ Inservice Educator
- g ☐ Field Nurse
- h ☐ Nursing Faculty
- j ☐ Nurse Clinician
- z ☐ Other _____
  specify

4. Hospital Nurses only:
- a ☐ Emergency Dept.
- b ☐ ICU/CCU
- c ☐ Medical/Surgical
- d ☐ Ob/Gyn/Nursery
- e ☐ Operating Room
- f ☐ Outpatient
- g ☐ Pediatrics
- h ☐ Psychiatric
- j ☐ Recovery Room
- k ☐ Anesthetist
- l ☐ Geriatrics
- m ☐ Central Service
- z ☐ Other Nursing Services

Special offer for new subscribers— $5 off Nursing81!

You'll learn about new developments and innovations—almost as soon as your colleagues perfect them! And follow their step-by-step solutions to the nursing problems *you* face every day.

You'll pick up useful tips and timesavers that will simplify… and *improve* your patient care. All in colorfully illustrated articles and features that really show you "how-to"!

☐ Send *Nursing81* for one year. My check for $15 is enclosed. (Saves me $5 off the published price!)   7S01

☐ Please bill me later.

Name _____

Address _____

City _____ State _____ Zip _____

Choose one of these important books as your introductory volume when you join the **NURSING SKILLBOOK** series...the most comprehensive reference series ever published for nurses.

- Using Crisis Intervention Wisely • Coping With Neurologic Problems Proficiently
- Managing Diabetics Properly • Helping Cancer Patients Effectively
- Documenting Patient Care Responsibly • Monitoring Fluid and Electrolytes Precisely • Giving Cardiovascular Drugs Safely • Assessing Vital Functions Accurately • Nursing Critically Ill Patients Confidently • Giving Emergency Care Competently • Reading EKGs Correctly • Combatting Cardiovascular Diseases Skillfully • Dealing with Death and Dying

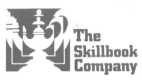
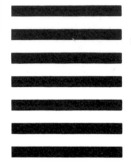

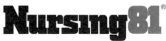
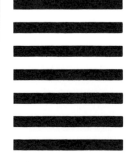

kidneys; he can become dehydrated. Be especially wary of dehydration in a patient who cannot complain of thirst.

The blood glucose level is usually lowered with regular insulin. Because patients with HHNK are not generally as insulin-resistant as DKA patients, and because they may have severe body fluid derangements, they usually should receive small and probably frequent doses. One more thing to watch for in patients whose metabolism has gotten out of hand: Their blood glucose level is quite labile. Monitor these patients closely, and watch the narrow line between soaring sugar levels and insulin shock.

Dehydration: Cause or effect?
No one seems sure whether dehydration leads to hyperosmolality—high concentration of solutes in the blood—or whether the hyperosmolality dehydrates by causing an osmotic diuresis, as it unmistakably does. No matter which, consider volume depletion and hyperosmolality together as the most serious part of HHNK, because they can lead directly to hypovolemic shock.

Under this threat, then, correcting both dehydration and hypertonicity is crucial. Logically, it would seem that hypotonic solutions would correct them fastest, and some authorities have recommended this. Yet it's safe to assume that through osmotic diuresis the patient has lost large total quantities not only of water, but of sodium, potassium, and accompanying anions—despite the probably high serum concentrations of those that remain. Consequently, the use of isotonic saline can help repair these absolute deficits. But, more importantly, it can do something else: It can help prevent a shift of water back into the intracellular fluid, whose relatively high concentration might otherwise withdraw the incoming water from the blood and perpetuate hyperosmolality.

Three-stage therapy
1. *Correct the sodium deficit* as rapidly as possible without overshooting the mark. Remember, many of these patients are elderly and may have heart disease. For Mr. Stevens, this correction consisted of 1 liter of normal saline over the first 2 hours.
2. *Correct the water deficit* rapidly, although incompletely. For this, use hypotonic fluid to rehydrate the patient and to

DPO 6

| Glucose mg/100 ml 720 |
| Serum acetone 0 |
| Urine acetone 0 |

BUN mg/100 ml 49
Sodium mEq/L 164
Potassium mEq/L 3.7
Chloride mEq/L 122
Total bilirubin mg/100 ml 14.1
Serum osmolality
   mosmol/Kg H_2O 378
Urine osmolality
   mosmol/Kg H_2O 755
Total protein GM/100 ml 5.1
PaO_2 mmHg 75
$PaCO_2$ 22.5
pH 7.53
HCO_3—mEq/L 18.4

DPO 8

| Glucose mg/100 ml 460 |
| Serum acetone 0 |
| Urine acetone 0 |

Sodium mEq/L 159
Potassium mEq/L 4.1
Chloride mEq/L 130
Total bilirubin mg/100 ml 8.6

DPO 13 DISCHARGE

| Glucose mg/100 ml 198 |
| Serum acetone 0 |
| Urine acetone 0 |

BUN mg/100 ml 49
Sodium mEq/L 148
Potassium mEq/L 3.1
Chloride mEq/L 108
Total protein GM/100 ml 5.1
PaO_2 mmHg 57.4
$PaCO_2$ 44.1
pH 7.38
HCO_3—mEq/L 21.5

DKA roadblock
Your treatment goals in managing patients with DKA are to:
• Clear serum and urine acetone
• Reduce blood sugar
• Correct dehydration and electrolyte imbalance
To achieve these goals, you must:
• Monitor vital signs, urine, and serum acetone.
• Maintain airway.
• Administer insulin as ordered.
• Relieve dehydration (I.V. infusion).
• Watch for signs of hypokalemia: leg cramps, weakness, nausea. Give plasma expander and multielectrolyte solution, as needed.

reduce hyperosmolality faster than added isotonic solution would do. The amount of hypotonic fluid needed by an individual to replace water deficit is based upon a comparison of effective and actual plasma osmolality.

When giving hypotonic solution, monitor the serum osmolality to prevent that shift of water back into the cells. Although 0.45% saline alone is often used for the hypotonic I.V. infusion, many doctors prefer fructose 2.5% in saline 0.45% until the blood sugar drops considerably. Fructose is rapidly absorbed from the blood, chiefly by the liver, and so does not contribute either to plasma tonicity or to osmotic diuresis. During the second stage of fluid therapy Mr. Stevens received 0.45% saline with 2.5% fructose and 5% dextrose in water.

3. *A cautious return to normal levels,* including electrolytes. On the eleventh postop day Mr. Stevens' potassium losses were great enough (serum potassium was down to 2.5 mEq/L) to require adding 60 mEq KCl/L to his I.V. infusion (amounting to 120 mEq/day). Of course, the serum electrolyte values don't always tell the true state of bodily derangement. For example, serum potassium levels can be high when the blood has borrowed potassium heavily from the cells, where nearly all of it is stored and used. But the kidneys can't conserve potassium well, so as soon as the blood's borrowed stores have been partly excreted, the patient will become hypokalemic. By this time the body may be critically short of its principal electrolyte. Serum potassium levels can also be high in HHNK when the patient is going into shock, so follow these serum values closely. But remember, they're only indicators, not absolutes.

Remember, glucocorticoids facilitate potassium shift. So Mr. Stevens' stressful condition and the hydrocortisone (Solu-Cortef) he received must have helped send potassium from cell to serum in the body's effort to keep the serum potassium levels normal—though they were then lowered by the continuing diuresis of hyperglycemia. Sodium is wasted by the diuresis, too, but proportionately more water is lost, so Mr. Stevens' hypernatremia primarily reflected dehydration.

Elevated blood urea nitrogen (BUN) is another common finding in patients with HHNK. Mr. Stevens' BUN rose after surgery from a normal 18 to the 50s. This increase in serum urea comes not only from dehydration, but often when there

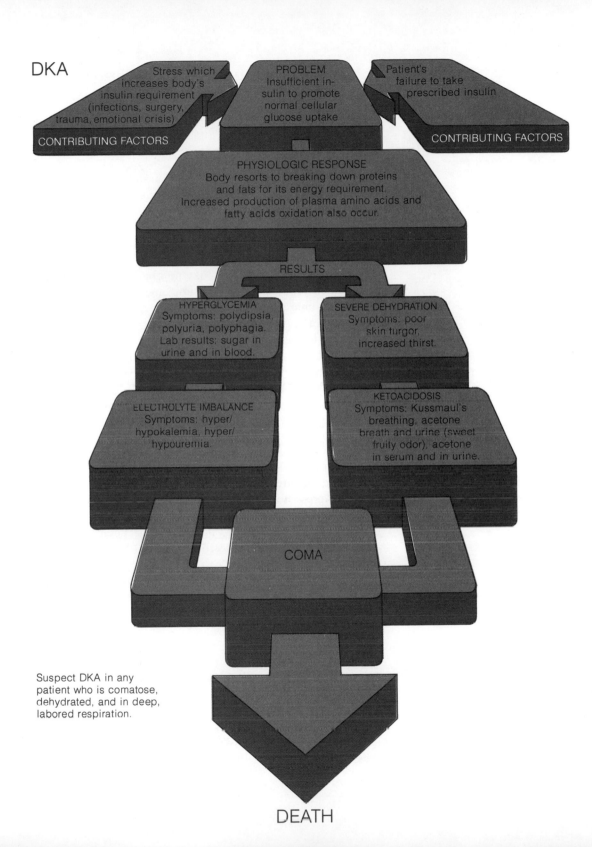

is stress or when glucocorticoids are given, from increased protein catabolism. And, incidentally, protein breakdown intensifies the loss of cellular potassium.

Nonketosis: The critical difference

Only the absence of ketoacidosis separates HHNK from a regular diabetic coma. When all the signs of DKA are there but this one—particularly when the glucose is elevated—that should alert you immediately to the true diagnosis.

What happens in DKA is this: The strongly acid ketones, including acetone, are formed, in the liver, out of mobilized fat. Normally, after suitable enzyme changes, they are oxidized by the tissues only for supplemental energy by the tissues and, unless insulin is lacking, they are formed no faster than they can be used. But without insulin (and so with glucose unavailable as energy to the cells), fats are called out in force and pile up in the blood as acetoacetic acid, a derivative, faster than coenzyme A can process it. In HHNK, on the other hand, the patient has enough insulin to avoid fat lipolysis and resultant ketoacidosis, but it is still too little to reduce hyperglycemia. The hyperglycemia, inducing diuresis, produces hyperosmolar blood, with no excessive production of ketone bodies and therefore no ketoacidosis.

It's also possible but still speculative that both glucocorticoids and dehydration have an antiketogenic effect. Glucocorticoids promote the synthesis of glucose from fats or from proteins (along with urea, raising the BUN). But, of course, glucose without insulin does not nourish the cells; it merely raises blood sugar, intensifies diuresis, and heightens hyperosmolality.

In HHNK, coma seems to result from both dehydration and hyperosmolality. Cerebral symptoms are probably due to fluid space and electrolyte derangements, and sometimes include seizures.

Preventing HHNK

• *Know your patient.* Be familiar with the pathophysiology of his medical problem so you can know when he runs a high risk of metabolic coma.

• *Maintain hydration.* To prevent dehydration, record intake and output scrupulously. Record daily weight, preferably on an in-bed scale. Notice the degree of skin turgor and mucosal moistness; loose skin and dry mouth are signs of dehydration. Hypotension and tachycardia are later signs of dehydration. You face particular problems with patients who can't complain of thirst, with elderly ones whose sense of thirst is dulled, and with those who are being hyperalimented or tube-fed. Make sure they get enough water. Usually, it's up to you to assess change and detect a need for fluid in any of these susceptible patients.

• *Keep a close check on sensorium.* Changes may be subtle, so it helps to have the same nursing staff care regularly for the patient in order to detect change more easily. Lethargy or confusion suggest a hyperosmolar state.

Treatment: Replacement and rehydration
During the first phase, replacement, when isotonic fluids are given rather rapidly to replace blood volume and sodium deficits, be sure the venous line is open and the flow rate is as ordered. Watch vital signs. *Stabilization of blood pressure will indicate restored volume.* During this period, measure urine output frequently.

During the second phase, rehydration, when the emphasis is on water replacement, you must be concerned about fluid overload, so monitor fluids very closely. Carefully control the rate of fluid administration. Be sure to check serum osmolality regularly and report any sudden or dramatic decrease to the doctor at once. Again, observe the sensorium. Its sudden deterioration might warn of cerebral edema.

Monitor glucose and acetone
Once you have identified your high-risk patients for HHNK, you can help protect them against it by monitoring the urine for glucose and acetone. A qualitative measurement of glucose provides the most accurate data. To get it, use a double-voided urine sample—one collected within an hour after the bladder has been emptied. This eliminates your reading any outdated glucose levels that might be present in residual urine.

We use reagent tablets such as Clinitest for glucose and Ketostix for acetone, q.i.d. (But remember that when the bilirubin is up or the patient is receiving cephalothin [Keflin], you may get a false positive and may have to fall back on Tes-Tape or Labstix.) Report blood glucose and urine tests on a regular schedule for consistent interpretation of results.

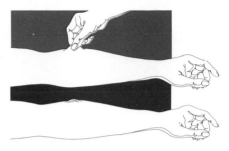

The pinch test
If you pinch the skin on a patient's forearm or sternum, under normal circumstances the skin will resume its shape quickly, within a few seconds. If the skin remains wrinkled for 20 to 30 seconds, however, the patient has poor skin turgor. Reduced or poor skin turgor may indicate dehydration, rapid weight reduction, or senile cutaneous atrophy. Report your findings to the doctor.

The definite difference

High blood glucose and glycosuria but no acetone, or only a trace, and no acidosis—these are what separate HHNK from diabetic ketoacidotic coma. (Lactic acidosis, another acidotic condition that can lead to coma, shows no acetone either, but, like DKA, it produces a low [acid] pH reading.)

Also remember the difference in treatment. In DKA, insulin is the key. Smaller amounts of fluid are needed to correct the correspondingly milder hyperosmolality of the blood. In HHNK, insulin is used sparingly; water is the key. Once the lost electrolytes are replaced with normal solutions, the quantities of hypotonic intravenous infusion also needed may bring the total fluids given to 10 or 20 liters during the first 48 hours. After hydration is resolved, insulin may be given more freely.

In fact, giving ample water may easily be the key to preventing this syndrome. All too often, when a patient's metabolic status is fluctuating—not only through imbalances of his own illness, but through the health team's continuous efforts to regulate them—something can go wrong. What goes wrong in HHNK is dehydration.

So keep alert for this among your susceptible patients— usually the elderly, the debilitated, and the mild or even unsuspected diabetic. Take the time to check their arms and legs for newly loosened skin, their face for a pinched look, and their tongue for dryness. After you have corrected dehydration, watch for another constant danger: water intoxication. For as soon as glucose levels are reduced, hyperosmolality of the blood is sharply reduced. This is when water is apt to be drawn into tissues, especially the brain. You can't watch for this too closely. If you keep the special characteristics of HHNK firmly in mind, you should be able to prevent hyperosmolar crisis.

13

DIC
Recognizing impending catastrophe

BY BONNIE MOWINSKI JENNINGS, RN, MSN

PERHAPS THE MOST DREADED complication in a critically ill patient is disseminated intravascular coagulation (DIC), a paradoxical combination of abnormal clotting and hemorrhage. You need to know how to recognize DIC in its earliest stages, before hemorrhage becomes severe and difficult to treat. Hazel Carter's case shows how suddenly DIC can become overwhelmingly severe...how difficult it can be to treat...and how important the right nursing care can be to survival.

Hazel Carter, a 30-year-old secretary, was hospitalized for evaluation of fever of unknown origin (FUO). Her relevant medical history began with diagnosis of collagen vascular disease in 1976. During the next 2 years, her condition worsened and was complicated by gastrointestinal intolerance to aspirin which was used to control fever, and combat joint inflammation and pain associated with collagen vascular disease.

At admission, Mrs. Carter's clotting tests were all within normal limits. During the second week of her extensive evaluation, an oral cholecystogram was done, followed by an intravenous pyelogram (IVP). A few hours later, she became short of breath and tachypneic. Suddenly, her blood pressure fell

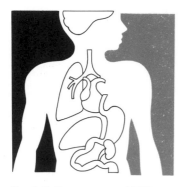

Precipitating causes of DIC
OBSTETRIC
Abruptio placentae
Retained dead fetus
Amniotic fluid embolism
Retained placenta
Toxemia
HEMOLYTIC
Transfusion of mismatched
blood
Acute hemolysis from infec-
tion or immunologic disorders
NECROTIC
Extensive burns and trauma
Rejection of transplants
Postoperative necrosis; espe-
cially following extracorporeal
circulation
NEOPLASTIC
Prostatic cancer
Acute leukemias
Giant cavernous hemangioma
Carcinoma
Sarcoma
INFECTIOUS
Acute bacteria
Virus
Fungus
Protozoa
Rickettsia
MISCELLANEOUS
Fat embolism
Snake bites
Glomerulonephritis
Thrombotic thrombocytopenia
purpura
Cirrhosis
Hypotension
Lung surgery
Heat stroke

from 105/60 to 80/60, and she became anxious and somewhat disoriented. Physical examination at this time revealed an acrocyanosis, sinus tachycardia of 130, and worsening tachypnea. Her blood pressure dropped to 50/0, and her pulse became thready — she was immediately transferred to the medical intensive care unit (MICU). There, a peripheral and a central intravenous line was placed for fluids and medication, and a Swan-Ganz catheter was placed to monitor pulmonary pressures and evaluate fluid status. Laboratory data revealed a hematocrit of 29%, hemopositive stools and nasogastric aspi-rate, and a creatinine level of 5.4 (normal to 1.5). Nasogastric bleeding cleared with iced saline lavage. Her known diagnoses at this time included acute tubular necrosis (ATN), shock of unclear etiology, early adult respiratory distress syndrome (ARDS), adult Still's disease, and gastrointestinal bleeding.

By morning of her second day in MICU, she continued to have respiratory distress. She had now developed a fever of 104° F. (40.0° C.), and a chest X-ray showed an infiltrate in the right lower lobe. Therefore, bronchoscopy was done to evaluate the possibility of pneumonia. The bronchoscopy re-sults were essentially normal, but soon after, Mrs. Carter began to bleed profusely from her nose. The blood flow was so profuse it obstructed her airway. She was therefore intubated orally and mechanical ventilation began. Anterior and pos-terior packs were placed in her nose to control the persistent nosebleed.

At this time, coagulation studies showed a marked deterio-ration from the previous day's results: prothrombin time was 15.7 (control, 11.3); prolonged partial thromboplastin time (PTT) was 54.0 (control, 33.0); and the platelet count was 59,000 (normal 150,000 to 400,000). Her fibrinogen had fallen from 213 mg per 100 ml at admission to MICU, to 50 mg per 100 ml. This blood picture confirmed DIC. Mrs. Carter clearly needed blood product replacement. Within 4 hours, she re-ceived 4 units of cryoprecipitate as a source of fibrinogen; 2 units of fresh frozen plasma to provide other clotting factors; and 2 units of packed red blood cells to counteract anemia from blood loss. These measures helped to diminish her bleeding to a slow ooze and were continued for 48 hours. However, even then her fibrinogen level persisted at a low 50 mg per 100 ml. So, her doctor decided to start continuous low-dose heparin infusion at 500 units per hour. With this, she showed dramatic improvement within 72 hours, her fibrin split products (FSPs) cleared, and the fibrinogen level and platelet count rose. Low-dose heparin infusion continued until her fibrinogen level exceeded 100 mg/100 ml and platelet count exceeded 100,000.

This patient with overwhelming DIC developed every possible difficulty with blood loss. Had you been in charge of Mrs. Carter's nursing care, would you have known how to proceed? How to give medications and personal care in ways that minimize the risk of additional bleeding? Would you have known how to recognize developing DIC before overt bleeding begins? What signs to look for in patients likely to develop DIC? To do all these things, you need to understand what actually happens in DIC. But first, you must understand normal coagulation...what is often called hemostasis.

How hemostasis happens

Normal hemostasis involves the interplay of the blood vessel wall, platelets, and the plasma proteins. In what is called primary hemostasis, arteriolar vasoconstriction occurs, then platelet aggregation forms a platelet plug at the site of bleeding.

Blood vessels react to injury with local vasoconstriction. This reaction presses endothelium together, enhances vessel wall stickiness and vessel adherence, which closes the vessel even after initial vasoconstriction subsides. When interstitial collagen from an injured blood vessel is exposed to circulating platelets, the collagen causes adhesiveness of platelets. These have the ability to stick to each other and to other surfaces to form clumps. When these platelets contact the torn, rough edges of the vessel wall they stick to the exposed collagen; they degranulate and release special substances (including platelet Factor III [a lipoprotein], and serotonin and epinephrine [necessary for coagulation]). At the same time, they release adenosine triphosphate (ADP). This substance increases platelet stickiness and facilitates their aggregation and the formation of a platelet plug.

For this mechanism to work properly, platelets must be present in the blood in sufficient numbers. What's sufficient? The normal count ranges from 150,000 to 400,000. Most hematologists agree that patients can have surgery without developing hemorrhage even with a platelet count as low as 50,000 if the platelets are in good condition. But with a platelet count between 30,000 and 20,000, spontaneous hemorrhage is

NORMAL CLOTTING

VASCULAR INJURY

Smooth-muscle spasm: serotonin is released

Vasoconstriction of blood vessels

Platelets adhering to rough surfaces of damaged vessels

ADP is released leading to further platelet breakdown

Loose platelet plug seals vessel wall and helps control bleeding

Fibrin threads form matrix

Fibrinogen is catalyzed to fibrin

Factor XIII (fibrin stabilizing factor) is activated

Platelets and blood cells are trapped in fibrin matrix, forming a blood clot

Factor XIII and calcium act on soluble fibrin to form a stable clot

Dissolution of fibrinolysis controls massive intravascular clotting

Clotting controls: Blood circulation removes excess thrombin; antithrombin II and III appear

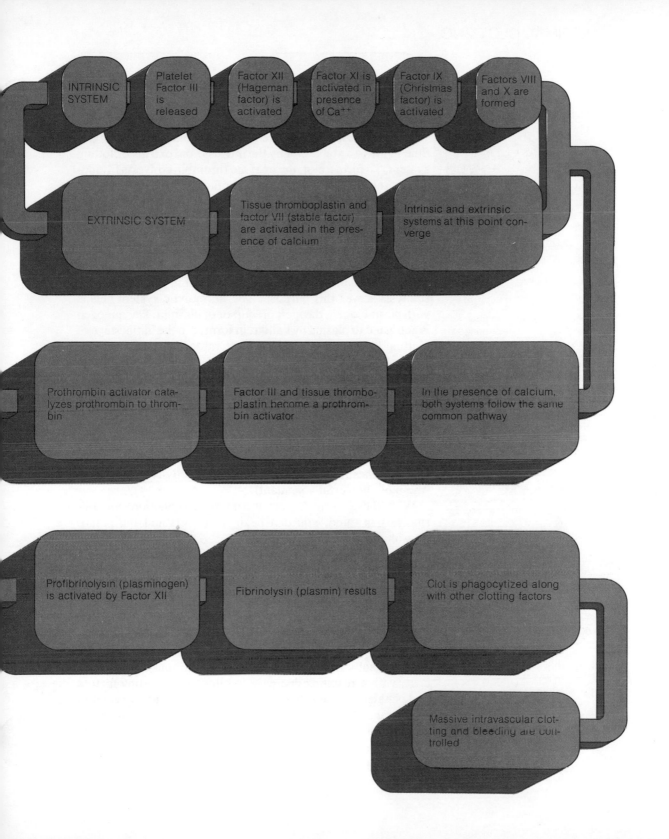

NURSING CRITICALLY ILL PATIENTS CONFIDENTLY

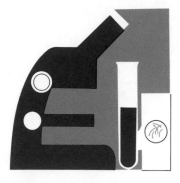

Lab values in DIC

Evaluation of plasma coagulation:
• Activated partial thrombo-plastin time (APTT)—prolonged: > 35 seconds.
• Partial thromboplastin time(PTT)—prolonged: > 60 to 90 seconds.
• Prothrombin time (PT)—prolonged: > 15 seconds.
• Thrombin time—prolonged: >15 to 20 seconds.
• Factor VIII assay—low.
• Factor V assay—low.
• Factor VII assay—low.

Evaluation of plasma fibrinogen levels:
• Fibrinogen level—low: < 75 mg/100 ml.
• Fibrin split products—ele-vated: > 100 mcg%.
• Euglobulin lysis test (fibrolytic activity)—shortened: < 12 minutes.

Evaluation of platelets:
• Platelet count—low: 75,000 to 20,000/mm3 of blood.
• Bleeding time (in vivo)—abnormal, prolonged: > 3 to 6 minutes (Duke) or > 3 to 7 minutes (IUY).
• Clotting time (in vitro)—prolonged: > 5 to 8 minutes.
• Peripheral smear—abnormal fragmented or helmet-shaped cells, instead of normal oval, disk-shaped cells.

likely; with a platelet count of only 10,000, intracerebral hemorrhage is possible.

After formation of the platelet plug, plasma proteins convert fluid blood to a stable clot by the intrinsic and extrinsic clotting system. To form a clot, the enzyme thrombin converts fibrinogen (a soluble plasma protein manufactured by the liver and normally present in the blood) into fibrin, an insoluble protein. Fibrin threads form a meshwork at the site of vessel injury, trapping red blood cells within, and thus forming a clot. The clot is then stabilized by plasma protein Factor XIII.

Obviously, if the coagulation process had no balancing counter mechanism, blood could not exist in fluid form. Fibrinolysis serves this purpose. The fibrinolytic system begins with plasminogen, the inert precursor of plasmin. Plasminogen is activated to plasma by kallikrein formed in the initial stage of clotting by Factor XII, plasma activators released from tissues, thrombin and other less clearly defined mechanisms. Also a part of this system are certain plasmin inhibitors and plasminogen activators, which are formed by the liver and which function as a complex, highly balanced system.

For additional protection against excessive clotting, the body forms antithrombins. The best known antithrombin responsible for anticoagulant activity is antithrombin III. As its name implies, antithrombin inhibits the activity of thrombin (the most powerful coagulant).

With these normal mechanisms of coagulation and fibrinolysis in mind, you can begin to understand the pathophysiology of DIC.

What is DIC?

DIC (disseminated intravascular coagulation) has been called by many other names: consumptive coagulopathy, defibrination syndrome, hypofibrinogenemia, and secondary fibrinolysis. However, DIC seems to be the most descriptive name. Lately, it's become the one most commonly used.

DIC results from acceleration of the normal clotting process, with a resulting decrease in circulating clotting factors and platelets. What actually happens in DIC? Fundamentally, a generalized activation of prothrombin, which produces an abundance of thrombin, which subsequently converts fibrinogen to fibrin and enhances platelet aggregation. This process consumes excessive amounts of many plasma proteins, especially fibrinogen, prothrombin, platelets Factor V and Factor VIII. Thus, patients with DIC develop hypofibrinogenemia, hypoprothrombinemia, and Factor V and Factor VIII deficiencies. As these factors are consumed, their concentration in the blood falls below the level needed for normal hemostasis; hemorrhage begins.

Remember that DIC is not a disease in itself but always a complication that develops as the aftermath of certain diseases and conditions. (See page 168 for list of disorders that may precipitate DIC.) Experts now believe that two basic mechanisms initiate DIC:

1) increased thromboplastin released from tissues such as the placenta, brain, and some tumors that activate the extrinsic system, and

2) activated Factor XII, which stimulates the intrinsic system (see pages 170-171, *Normal Clotting*).

DIC begins when excessive or accelerated intravascular thrombin converts fibrinogen to a fibrin clot and enhances platelet aggregation. This consumes clotting factors and platelets to the point of depletion. Such depletion makes clotting impossible and predisposes to hemorrhage.

How to detect DIC?

Suspect developing DIC when you find abnormal bleeding in a patient with no previous serious bleeding history. The bleeding may vary from mild oozing at venipuncture sites to hemorrhage from all orifices (the latter is common in full-blown DIC). Other signs may also point to developing DIC: acrocyanosis (cyanosis of the digits) or peripheral thrombosis.

You can't be absolutely sure a patient has DIC until you have confirmed the depletion of circulation clotting factors through certain laboratory tests. These tests identify DIC by measuring the circulating levels of clotting factors and platelets. In a patient with overt or developing DIC, you'll find prolonged prothrombin time; prolonged partial thromboplastin time; prolonged thrombin time; decreased fibrinogen levels; and decreased platelet count. If all of these tests are normal, no significant DIC exists. But even if they are clearly abnormal, further testing may be needed to confirm DIC.

Three special laboratory tests are diagnostic for DIC: fibrin split products (FSPs), protamine sulfate, and specific factors analysis. Patients with DIC have elevated levels of fibrin split products. As a great many clots are formed, so are a correspondingly greater number of breakdown products from the degradation of fibrin and fibrinogen. FSPs work three ways to inhibit blood coagulation:

• They coat the platelets and so diminish their adhesivity.

• They inhibit the powerful coagulant, thrombin.

• They attach to fibrinogen (which inhibits polymerization, a process necessary to form a stable clot).

Perhaps the most sensitive test for DIC is the protamine sulfate test. Protamine sulfate can bind with fibrin split products and free the fibrin monomer so it can be polymerized and form a stable clot. A weakly positive test is possible in patients with liver disease or thrombosis, or patients who have recently had surgery. However, a strongly positive test is highly indicative of DIC. The last special test assesses the patient's plasma for certain plasma protein factors suspected to be deficient in DIC. Factor assays may be done to determine the exact amounts of these factors present.

Management difficult

Successful management of DIC requires that you and the doctors recognize it promptly; correctly and vigorously treat the underlying disease; and combat DIC itself.

Recognizing DIC promptly requires you to watch for the subtlest signs of abnormal bleeding. First of all, remember that blood loss causes anemia. So don't overlook a patient's unexplained complaints of fatigue, weakness, myalgia, or malaise. Visual inspection may be your best source of clues to DIC. Examine the patient's skin and mucous membranes for pallor, purpura, and jaundice. Also check his conjunctivae and sclerae for icterus and hemorrhage. Be alert for complaints of blurred or impaired vision, which might suggest retinal hemorrhage.

Nosebleeds are dramatic and impossible to overlook — unless the bleeding is from the posterior nasopharynx. You might overlook such bleeding because the patient may swallow the blood. This kind of bleeding has sometimes led to fatal hemorrhage, so keep this possibility in mind. Gingival bleeding may be a sign of DIC. Remember that changing mentation may also be a sign of cerebral bleeding. Such changes may range from headaches and vertigo to irritability and confusion.

Once overt bleeding begins, the patient will begin to show

CLOTTING MECHANISM IN DIC

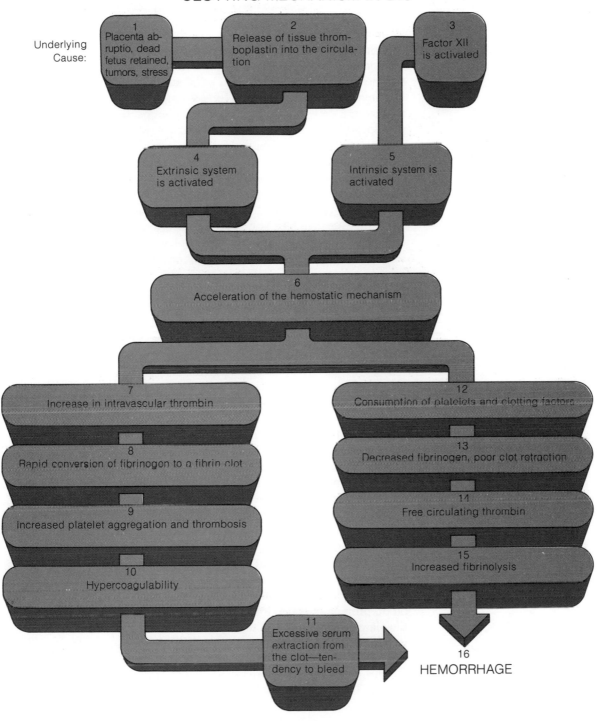

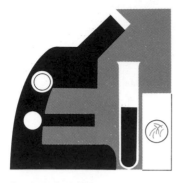

Coagulation tests
To assess clotting potential and follow the effects of anticoagulant treatment, several tests are used:
Bleeding time (Duke) depends on the number and functional activity of platelets, the prothrombin content of the blood, the ability of tissue factors to initiate clotting, and the vessels' response to rupture. It is therefore a measure of the body's ability to seal a small wound.
Coagulation time (Lee-White) measures the time interval between the appearance of blood in a siliconized syringe and the clotting of blood. Normal coagulation time is 3 to 8 minutes.
Prothrombin time (Quick) is the coagulation time obtained when an excess of thromboplastin and calcium is added to oxalated plasma under standardized conditions. Normal prothrombin time is 12 to 17 seconds. This is increased in persons with prothrombin deficiency or deficiencies of Factors V, VII, and X.

systemic symptoms of abnormal cardiopulmonary status. As his body tries to maintain adequate cardiac output to oxygenate the tissues, you'll find him developing tachypnea, orthopnea, tachycardia, murmurs, palpitations, and orthostatic hypotension. If bleeding continues long enough to cause myocardial deficit, he may develop angina pectoris; or if he develops bleeding within the lungs, he'll have hemoptysis.

Learn to recognize subtle signs of abdominal bleeding. For example, retroperitoneal bleeding may not cause abdominal tenderness, but instead may cause numbness and pain in a leg (because of compression of the lateral femoral cutaneous nerve in the region of L1 to L3). You know that hematemesis points to intestinal bleeding as do melenic (upper GI bleeding) and hematochezic (lower GI) stools. Of course, you also need to watch for gross or occult hematuria, the result of genitourinary bleeding.

Bone tenderness and joint pain may also be important symptoms of DIC. The bone tenderness and pain result from infarctions caused by fibrin clots.

Treating the underlying disease that led to DIC might be a simple matter of supportive measures during self-limiting conditions. More likely, though, the cause of DIC needs highly specific and dramatic therapy. In every case, however, correctly treating the primary disease is essential to overcome DIC.

Combatting DIC itself is considerably more difficult than recognizing it and treating its causes. Researchers are still looking for the best way to combat full-blown DIC. Currently, treatment varies, depending on severity.

In a patient who isn't bleeding, DIC needs no specific treatment. Just treating the underlying disease may reverse the DIC. However, once the patient has begun to bleed, treatment must also include measures that specifically support hemostasis — the administration of supplementary platelets and clotting factors. If the patient continues unimproved after vigorous treatment of the underlying disease combined with blood product support, intravenous heparin may be added to the platelet and clotting factor replacement. The use of heparin is somewhat controversial. However, its proponents believe that heparin's antithrombin activity neutralizes free circulating thrombin, thereby preventing proliferation of thrombi in the capillaries, and inhibiting blood clotting. Heparin must always be used with platelet and clotting factor replacement.

Nursing management complex

Nursing management of patients with DIC has two components: compensation for anemia and prevention of additional bleeding.

Nursing care for the patient who has lost or hemolyzed large numbers of red blood cells must compensate for the resulting anemia. Such anemia means an inadequate number of erythrocytes available to transport oxygen to the cells via hemoglobin, and to maintain acid-base balance through the buffering action of hemoglobin. Therefore, care of a severely anemic patient has to provide for rest, which will help to decrease tissue and myocardial oxygen demands, and carefully monitor orthostatic vital signs, cardiopulmonary status, and arterial blood gases. Specifically, you must plan patient care to alternate periods of activity and rest (thereby decreasing oxygen requirements). Explain to the patient why he might feel unusual fatigue or weakness. If blood loss is severe enough to reduce the vascular fluid volume necessary for maintaining blood pressure, move the patient slowly when changing his position, and monitor intravenous fluid infusions carefully.

To monitor cardiopulmonary status, you must go beyond observable symptoms such as dyspnea and tachycardia: Check the hemoglobin content and results of blood-gas analysis for acid-base balance, oxygen saturation, and potential hypoxemia. Remember, the patient with anemia can be hypoxic and have normal blood-gas values. Hemoglobin carries oxygen to the tissues. Blood gases measure only the oxygen that is dissolved in the plasma. If hemoglobin is available to remove oxygen from the plasma and deliver it to the tissues, tissue hypoxia results even though there is an adequate supply of oxygen within the circulatory system. The patient with hypoxemia needs red blood cell replacement. Correcting hypoxemia is essential because hypoxemia may lead to acidemia; acidemia may aggravate DIC.

To care for such patients competently, you must know the best techniques for administering blood product replacement. You want to offer maximum benefit from blood replacement with minimal side effects. Some important considerations for giving blood products safely include: *accurate* patient and product identification; infusion of product with normal saline; use of blood tubing with a filter; use of a large enough needle at the venipuncture site; and proper monitoring of vital signs before, during, and after administration.

Prevent additional bleeding

First, of course, you must observe common bleeding sites to detect hemorrhage early and quickly intervene. For example, if the patient has a nosebleed, it's helpful to put the patient in high-Fowler's position to prevent aspiration of blood. Such a patient also needs something to control the bleeding (nose clips, ice packs, nasal packing, or ice). To discover overt GI and genitourinary bleeding, routinely guaic-test all stools or emesis, and hematest all urine. Finally, be alert for changes in the patient's mental status because irritability and confusion can indicate intracranial hemorrhaging.

Monitor your nursing techniques to prevent breaks in skin that can serve as additional bleeding sites. Consider this when giving personal care. For example, avoid nicks and cuts by using an electric razor to shave male patients. When giving mouth care, reduce friction on the gums in every way you can: baby-bristle toothbrushes; cotton swabs; mild mouthwash; or a Water Pik, which might be less abrasive than other mouth-care elements. To get back to Mrs. Carter — she had gingival oozing, so we gave her the gentlest mouth care with warm water and cotton swabs, being careful not to dislodge any clots that had formed on her gums.

Avoid intramuscular and subcutaneous administration of medications whenever possible. In patients with DIC, these routes often cause hematomas. However, if intramuscular or subcutaneous injections are absolutely unavoidable, use a very small-gauge needle and, immediately afterward, apply pressure at the puncture site for as long as necessary — several minutes at least. Use the same technique for controlling bleeding from venipuncture and intravenous sites.

Mrs. Carter needed many medications. We injected them through existing intravenous lines, rather than through intramuscular or subcutaneous routes that could have become additional bleeding sites. Obviously, some venipunctures were unavoidable to place and change intravenous lines and to procure blood specimens. Mrs. Carter did, in fact, develop some purpura and hematomas secondary to these venipunctures, but to keep the hematomas as small as possible, her nurses applied pressure at the puncture sites for 5 to 10 minutes, until oozing stopped, each time they had to start an I.V. infusion or blood replacement.

If the patient has any catheters or tubes inserted through his nose (such as nasal prongs for oxygen, nasogastric suction, or a nasotracheal tube) try to prevent irritation or breakdown of the skin. During tracheal suctioning, take care not to traumatize the mucosa because serious bleeding difficulties may follow.

Since epistaxis was a major problem for Mrs. Carter, we had to carefully evaluate bleeding from the posterior nasopharynx. We reported and recorded any bloody aspirate suctioned from her mouth or throat. Similarly, we monitored oozing through the nasal packing. When washing her face, we took care to avoid dislodging any clots that had formed on the outside of the nasal packing. Since her oral tracheal tube and, later, her tracheostomy were foci for irritation, skin breakdown, and bleeding, we watched these areas carefully. We carefully inspected the tracheal aspirate to assure that suctioning had not traumatized the mucosa to establish another site for bleeding.

Also prevent trauma

You can protect the patient with DIC from trauma in many ways. During blood pressure readings, pressure from the cuff can break superficial capillaries and produce purpura. To prevent this, it may help to: use a different extremity for blood pressure reading (in rotational order); avoid overinflating the cuff; take blood pressure readings only when necessary; and do the readings quickly.

To *minimize the number of cuff pressures* necessary in Mrs. Carter, we monitored blood pressure through the use of an arterial line. (We used cuff pressures only to validate the accuracy of the monitor pressures.) We also used the arterial line to acquire blood specimens, which helped to reduce the number of venipunctures. However, because we had to infuse heparin through the arterial line to maintain its patency, we drew blood specimens for coagulation studies from another site (thereby eliminating heparin as a contaminant of the tests).

Practice environmental safety to avoid hematomas from injury. For example, pad the side rails of the bed for a patient who is confused or having seizures. Continually observe for purpura. Also, remember to warn the hemorrhaging patient against straining during bowel movements. Straining against a

**Common
A.S.A.-containing products**
Alka-Seltzer Effervescent
   Pain Reliever and Antacid
Anacin
Arthritis Strength Bufferin
A.S.A. Compound
   Capsules
Ascriptin
Aspergum
   (gum tablet)
Bufferin
Cope
Empirin Compound
Excedrin
Excedrin P.M.
Sine-Aid
Vanquish Caplet

PRESCRIPTION AND
NONPRESCRIPTION
PRODUCTS CONTAINING A.S.A.
A.P.C.
Darvon Compound-65
Darvon with A.S.A.
Empirin
Equagesic
P-A-C Compound
Talwin Compound

OTC-A.S.A.-CONTAINING PRODUCTS
COLD, ALLERGY MEDICATIONS
Alka-Seltzer Plus
Bayer Decongestant
Congespirin
Coricidin
Coricidin D
Dristan
Sine-Off
4-Way Cold Tablets

SLEEP-AID/SEDATIVE
Quiet World Tablets

closed glottis can raise blood pressure high enough to rupture a blood vessel.

Consider the effects of aspirin. Aspirin interferes with platelet aggregation, further inhibiting coagulation. Consequently, avoid all aspirin and aspirin-containing products in any patient who has DIC. Remember, innumerable medications contain aspirin even though their names don't make this obvious (see insert).

Know how to give blood products correctly. When replacing clotting factors and platelets, you must understand just how each component can help the patient. For example, you need to know that fresh frozen plasma replaces clotting factors and provides a source of antithrombin; platelet support is indicated for low platelet counts; and cryoprecipitate is a concentrated preparation which contains fibrinogen and Factor VIII. The techniques for giving these blood products are essentially the same as for red blood cell replacement. But remember one difference that relates to platelets: Keep platelets at room temperature. The other blood components need refrigeration.

Measure the amount of blood lost. This means weighing bandages and linen, recording drainage, and counting the number of sanitary napkins used. Also remember that internal blood loss, especially as hematomas, will also deplete vascular volume. Measure the extremities of the abdomen for enlargement which may help to document internal blood loss. Assessing blood loss accurately helps you to refine management. It allows you to measure fluid and blood replacement precisely; to evaluate and modify treatment; and to monitor the progress of the DIC.

Caring for patients with DIC is difficult indeed and challenges all your knowledge and nursing skill. The correct application of these nursing skills, no less than medical treatment, is critical to the patient's survival.

SKILLCHECK 3

1. You're caring for 17-year-old Ned Perfetti, who's in traction for a fractured femur he acquired in a skiing accident. Two days after the accident, Ned develops a fever and becomes cyanotic and agitated. You also notice a rash on his chest and shoulders. What do these signs indicate?
a) Shock
b) Fat embolism
c) Sepsis
d) Pneumonia.

2. Mr. Savas, a 45-year-old engineer with no previous cardiac history, returns to your unit after an exploratory laporotomy. Although other assessments are within normal limits, his pulse is 130. Is this a normal finding? Why is it, or isn't it?

3. Two hours after 58-year-old Mr. Allen arrives in the recovery room following a right inguinal hernia repair under spinal anesthesia, you note that his blood pressure is 90 over 48. He has some sensation in his legs but can't yet move them, he hasn't voided, and he's restless and complaining of pain. What might be causing his hypotension?
a) Pain
b) Urinary retention
c) Anesthesia
d) All the above.

4. Mr. Shaw was admitted to your unit for evaluation because of a history of passing black, tarry stools. About an hour after admission he suddenly vomits about 500 ml of bright red blood. What might his emesis indicate?
a) Low gastrointestinal bleeding
b) Old bleeding—the blood has been in contact with gastric juices for several hours.
c) Bleeding somewhere above the ligament of Treitz.
d) All the above.

5. Which of the following is *not* a goal of therapy for Mr. Shaw or for any other GI bleeder?
a) Maintaining blood volume and tissue perfusion
b) Assessing and controlling bleeding
c) Avoiding complications
d) Beginning sterold therapy.

6. Propranolol (Inderal) is useful in the treatment of

thyrotoxicosis because it:
a) Reduces the plasma thyroxine concentration
b) Prevents congestive heart failure
c) Controls the tachycardia, tremors, and nervousness associated with thyrotoxicosis
d) Is known to cause hypothyroidism.

7. In which of the following situations should an adrenally insufficient patient increase his corticosteroid dose?
a) Dental extraction
b) Fractured femur
c) Surgery
d) Flu
e) All the above.

8. The major clinical manifestation of HHNK is:
a) Blood glucose level above 600 mg per 100 ml
b) Serum hypo-osmolality
c) Acidemia
d) Ketonuria.

9. Which of the following conditions increases a patient's risk of developing HHNK?
a) Diabetes mellitus
b) Cortisone therapy for arthritis
c) Pancreatitis
d) Extensive burns
e) All the above.

10. You're caring for Mrs. Wisniewski, an elderly appendectomy patient. Five days after surgery her temperature jumps to 104° F. (40° C.). The next day she begins bleeding from venipuncture sites, although she has no previous history of abnormal bleeding. Subsequent evaluation reveals diffuse bronchopneumonia. Can you identify her problem?
a) Disseminated intravascular coagulation (DIC)
b) Thyroid storm
c) Encephalopathy
d) Hepatitis.

11. Which of the following is *not* a screening test for disseminated intravascular coagulation (DIC)?
a) PT
b) Hematocrit and hemoglobin
c) PTT
d) Platelet count.

(Answers on page 184)

SKILLCHECK ANSWERS

ANSWERS TO SKILLCHECK 1 (Page 35)

Situation 1
The three parts of your nursing assessment should include:
a) Mrs. Tyler's history and her family history
b) A physical examination, including inspection, palpation, auscultation, and percussion
c) Laboratory data.

Situation 2
d) *Use of tapping to elicit vibrations.*

Situation 3
c) *May cause abnormalities in mental function lasting up to 10 days.* Sedatives may in fact disturb the normal sleep cycle, and allowing 30-minute sleep periods without interruption won't permit the completion of a normal sleep cycle, which lasts from 80 to 120 minutes.

Situation 4
a) *Psychologic stress.* If left unchecked, psychologic stress may contribute to other conditions, such as the inability to sleep, which could possibly lead to hallucinations or delirium.

Situation 5
d) *Intestinal gas.* A loud, bell-like sound of variable pitch indicates the presence of air or gas in a body cavity.

Situation 6
c) *Press down with your fingertips.* In deep palpation, you would use the heel of your hand, or you could even use both hands.

Situation 7
Discourage pregelling the defibrillator. This is a sloppy procedure, since the gel dries and cakes unless it's used immediately. Then it has to be scraped off and a fresh layer must be applied before the defibrillator is used, or the patient may suffer electrical burns. Ultimately, this procedure takes more time than starting from scratch and may endanger a patient's life in an emergency.

Situation 8
b) *Include him in decision-making and avoid restraining him.* Mr. Freitas' independent behavior is his way of coping with his illness and the frightening ICU environment, both of which make him feel helpless. Restraining him or threatening to restrain him will only increase his anxiety. Sedating him will alter his senses and may make the ICU seem even more frightening. It may also interfere with his breathing, which is already compromised.

ANSWERS TO SKILLCHECK 2 (Page 99)

Situation 1
c) *20 g daily.* This provides enough essential amino acids for tissue repair and maintenance. It is also sufficient to avoid a negative nitrogen balance resulting from catabolism of the body's own tissue.

Situation 2
c) *It's the most rapid and efficient method of dialysis.* This statement is true of hemodialysis, but not peritoneal dialysis. Peritoneal dialysis takes from 48 to 72 hours, while hemodialysis takes only 3 to 4 hours.

Situation 3
c) *Vasoconstrictors.* Giving a vasoconstrictor *would* increase blood pressure, but it would also markedly increase the heart's workload and contribute to pump failure. A diuretic is useful to remove excess fluid, and a vasodilator reduces both preload and afterload, thereby decreasing the workload of the heart.

Situation 4
d) *Call the doctor immediately to reposition the catheter.* It has slipped out of the pulmonary artery and into the right ventricle, and should be repositioned immediately to avoid ventricular fibrillation.

Situation 5
d) *Pleural effusion.* Both these sounds point to fluid in the pleural space.

Situation 6
b) *Bradycardia and widening pulse pressure.* But don't use these signs as indicators of increased intracranial

pressure—by the time they're present, permanent brain damage may have occurred.

Situation 7
d) *All the above*.

Situation 8
a) *All may cause blood ammonia levels to rise, leading to hepatic encephalopathy*.

Situation 9
a) *Administration of a diuretic*. This may in fact, increase Mrs. D'Onofrio's potassium loss. Preventing nausea, vomiting, and diarrhea, and administering a potassium supplement will all help reduce her potassium deficiency.

ANSWERS TO SKILLCHECK 3
Situation 1
b) *Fat embolism*. Ned's rash is the distinguishing sign of this complication.

Situation 2
When all other signs are normal, increased heart rate postoperatively is usually nothing to worry about. It's a normal compensatory mechanism to maintain cardiac output at a level sufficient to meet tissue oxygen needs. The rate will most likely diminish without treatment as these needs are met.

Situation 3
d) *All the above*. To help Mr. Allen, raise his legs to promote venous return and to augment circulating volume, check for bladder distention and obtain an order for catheterization if it's present, and give a partial dose of an analgesic to relieve pain.

Situation 4
c) *Bleeding somewhere above the ligament of Treitz*. If blood has been in contact with gastric juices for

several hours, it becomes dark in color or like coffee grounds. Lower GI bleeding doesn't usually cause vomiting.

Situation 5
d) *Beginning steroid therapy*. Steroids may *cause* GI bleeding.

Situation 6
c) *Controls the tachycardia, tremors, and nervousness associated with thyrotoxicosis*. Propranolol (Inderal) is a beta adrenergic blocker that prevents increased sympathetic nervous system activity.

Situation 7
e) *All the above*. During all periods of stress, adrenally insufficient patients should increase their corticosteroid dose. This simulates what occurs normally in patients with a functioning hypothalamic-pituitary-adrenal axis.

Situation 8
a) *Blood glucose level above 600 mg per 100 ml*. In HHNK the serum is hyperosmolar, and acidemia and ketonuria aren't present.

Situation 9
e) *All the above*. These conditions all increase the risk of hyperglycemia, and this is a forerunner of HHNK.

Situation 10
a) *Disseminated intravascular coagulation (DIC)*. Abnormal bleeding from Mrs. Wisniewski's venipuncture sites should lead you to suspect that her clotting factors are depleted.

Situation 11
b) *Hematocrit and hemoglobin*. PT, PTT, and a platelet count can all point to the decrease in circulating clotting factors and platelets typical of DIC.

GLOSSARY

autodigestion—autolysis; the digestion of the body's own tissues by its own secretions.

azotemia—an excess of urea or other nitrogenous products in the bloodstream due to renal insufficiency.

chest tubes, milking—fold tubing and squeeze repeatedly to loosen material that has collected on sides.

chest tubes, stripping—hold tubing at top with one hand, at same time squeezing tube and pulling downward with other hand to express fluid and maintain an unobstructed flow.

colloid—a substance which remains suspended in a solution, neither dissolving nor settling.

corneal reflex—normal response to stimulation of the cornea causing eye to blink; absence of this response denotes injury, coma, or nerve injury.

crepitus—crackling movement heard on auscultation or felt on palpation, usually due to air, gas, or fragments of bone.

fremitus—vibration or thrill detected during auscultation or palpation.

granuloma—well-defined node of granulomatous tissue formed after prolonged inflammation due to infectious disease or foreign body.

hemoconcentration—erythrocyte concentration appears to have increased, but is due to a decrease in plasma, not an increase in erythrocytes. Found in shock, burns, and diabetes mellitus.

hyperosmotic—solution containing a high concentration of compounds.

hypoxic shock—occurs in all types of shock when available oxygen is insufficient to meet body needs. When oxygen need continues to be greater than that available, tissue death occurs and shock becomes irreversible.

icterus—jaundice; raised bilirubin levels in blood, producing yellowish appearance of skin, sclera, and mucous membranes.

ileus—intestinal obstruction usually caused by partial muscular paralysis causing absence of peristalsis in the affected area.

IMV—(intermittent mandatory ventilation) permits the patient to breathe spontaneously with any pattern and tidal volume he desires, without assistance by the respirator. A preset volume of gas will be delivered to the patient at regular intervals at a preset frequency.

Korotkoff's sounds—sounds heard in the brachial artery when systolic blood pressure level is reached. They occur simultaneously with each pulse beat, becoming muffled at the diastolic level and disappearing entirely after that.

Kupffer's cells—large, intensely phagocytic cells that line the walls of the sinusoids of the liver; part of the reticuloendothelial system.

palmar erythema—redness of the palms of the hands due to capillary dilatation caused by injury, inflammation, or infection.

PEEP—(positive end expiratory pressure). A positive pressure maintained at the airway opening throughout the respiratory cycle. This pressure, usually 5 to 10 cm H_2O, prevents the collapse of small airways during exhalation and improves the distribution of gases throughout the lungs.

pleurisy—inflammation of the lining of the chest cavity (pleural). Dry pleurisy is characterized by pain on inhalation and friction rub; wet pleurisy by distention on the affected site and absence of breathing movement.

proptosis—(exophthalmos) a bulging or forward displacement of one or both eyeballs. Usually due to orbital inflammation, or in thyrotoxicosis, edema, tumors, or injuries.

pyelolithotomy—the surgical removal of renal calculi from the kidney.

rigor—sudden chill accompanied by severe shivering, followed by profuse perspiration; also rigidity.

spider angiomas—vascular tumor produced by capillary dilatation from which small blood vessels radiate resembling a spider's web.

Still's disease—a form of rheumatoid arthritis presenting as fever of unknown origin, with joint aches and rash; mainly found in children, but can also occur in adults.

SUGGESTED FURTHER READING

Bates, Barbara. A GUIDE TO PHYSICAL EXAMINATION. Philadelphia, J.B. Lippincott Company, 1974.

Beland, Irene L., and Joyce Y. Passos. CLINICAL NURSING. 3rd ed. New York, Macmillan Publishing Co., Inc., 1975.

Brundage, Dorothy J. NURSING MANAGEMENT OF RENAL PROBLEMS. St. Louis, C.V. Mosby Company, 1976.

Brunner, Lillian S., and Doris S. Suddarth. THE LIPPINCOTT MANUAL OF NURSING PRACTICE. 2nd ed. Philadelphia, J.B. Lippincott Company, 1978.

Brunner, Lillian S., et al. TEXTBOOK OF MEDICAL-SURGICAL NURSING. 3rd ed. Philadelphia, J.B. Lippincott Company, 1975.

Burrell, Zeb L., and Lenette Owens Burrell. CRITICAL CARE. 3rd ed. St. Louis, C.V. Mosby Company, 1977.

Byers, Virginia B. NURSING OBSERVATION. 2nd ed. Foundations of Nursing Series. Dubuque IA, William C. Brown Publishing Company, 1977.

Conn, Howard, ed. CURRENT THERAPY 1978. Philadelphia, W.B. Saunders Company, 1978.

DuGas, Beverly W. KOZIER-DU GAS' INTRODUCTION TO PATIENT CARE. 3rd ed. Philadelphia, W.B. Saunders Company, 1977.

Hamburger, Joel I. CLINICAL EXERCISES IN INTERNAL MEDICINE:Thyroid disease, Vol. 1. Philadelphia, W.B. Saunders Company, 1978.

Hoffman, William S. THE BIOCHEMISTRY OF CLINICAL MEDICINE. 4th ed. Chicago, Year Book Medical Publishers, 1970.

Hudak, Carolyn M., Thelma Lohr, and Barbara M. Gallo. CRITICAL CARE NURSING. 2nd ed. Philadelphia, J.B. Lippincott Company, 1977.

Krueger, Judith A., and Janis C. Ray. ENDOCRINE PROBLEMS IN NURSING: A physiologic approach. St. Louis, C.V. Mosby Company, 1976.

Krupp, Marcus A., and Milton J. Chatton, eds. CURRENT MEDICAL DIAGNOSIS AND TREATMENT 1978. Los Altos CA, Lange Medical Publications, 1978.

Luckmann, Joan, and Karen Sorensen. MEDICAL-SURGICAL NURSING:A psychophysiologic approach. Philadelphia, W.B. Saunders Company, 1974.

MacLeod, John. DAVIDSON'S PRINCIPLES AND PRACTICE OF MEDICINE. 12th ed. New York, Churchill Livingstone,1978.

Rose, Leslie I., and Robert L. Lavine. NEW CONCEPTS IN ENDOCRINOLOGY AND METABOLISM:39th Hahnemann Symposium on endocrinology and metabolism. New York, Grune and Stratton, 1977.

Secor, Jane. PATIENT CARE IN RESPIRATORY PROBLEMS. Monographs in Clinical Nursing:Vol. 1. Philadelphia, W.B. Saunders Company, 1969.

Werner, Sidney C., and Sidney H. Ingbar. THE THYROID. 4th ed. Hagerstown MD, Harper and Row, 1978.

Williams, Robert H. TEXTBOOK OF ENDOCRINOLOGY. 5th ed. Philadelphia, W.B. Saunders Company, 1974.

Wintrobe, Maxwell M., ed., et al. HARRISON'S PRINCIPLES OF INTERNAL MEDICINE. 8th ed. New York, McGraw-Hill Book Company, 1977.

Wright, Samson, ed. SAMSON WRIGHT'S APPLIED PHYSIOLOGY. 12th ed. New York, Oxford University Press, 1971.

INDEX